Pro

MW00903848

Richard K. Johns MD

Steven E. Armstrong

Water Balance in Schizophrenia

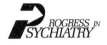

Number 48

**David Spiegel, M.D.
Series Editor**

Water Balance in Schizophrenia

Edited by David B. Schnur, M.D., and Darrell G. Kirch, M.D.

Published by

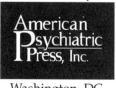

Washington, DC
London, England

Copyright © 1996 American Psychiatric Press, Inc.

ALL RIGHTS RESERVED

Manufactured in the United States of America on acid-free paper

First Edition   98   97   96   95   4   3   2   1

American Psychiatric Press, Inc.
1400 K Street, N.W., Washington, DC   20005

Library of Congress Cataloging-in-Publication Data
Water balance in schizophrenia / edited by David B. Schnur, Darrell G.
  Kirch.
        p. cm.—(Progress in psychiatry series; #48)
     Includes bibliographical references and index.
     ISBN 0-88048-485-3
     1. Schizophrenia—Pathophysiology. 2. Water-electrolyte imbalances.
  I. Schnur, David B., 1949-   . II. Kirch, Darrell G., 1949-   . III. Series.
     [DNLM: 1. Schizophrenia—physiopathology. 2. Water-Electrolyte
  Balance. W1 PR6781L no. 48 1996 / WM 203 W324 1996]
RC514.W26 1996
616.89'8207—dc20
DNLM/DLC
for Library of Congress
                                                              95-46598
                                                                  CIP

British Library Cataloguing in Publication Data
A CIP record is available from the British Library.

Contents

Contributors

Carla Canuso, M.D.
Chief Resident, Department of Psychiatry, University of Chicago, Chicago, Illinois

Ahmed M. Elkashef, M.D.
Senior Staff Fellow, Neuropsychiatry Branch, National Institute of Mental Health, Neuroscience Center at St. Elizabeths Hospital, Washington, D.C.

Morris B. Goldman, M.D.
Associate Professor of Psychiatry, and Director of Research, Psychiatric Institute, Department of Psychiatry, University of Chicago, Chicago, Illinois

Sebastian P. Grossman, Ph.D.
Professor, Department of Biological Psychology, University of Chicago, Chicago, Illinois

Jon R. Hammersberg, M.D.
Attending Physician, Western State Hospital, Staunton, Virginia

Patricia B. Higgens, L.C.S.W., M.S.W.
Clinical Social Work Supervisor, University of Virginia, Department of Psychiatry, Western State Hospital, Staunton, Virginia

Barbara Illowsky Karp, M.D.
Chief, Neurology Consultation Service and Assistant Clinical Director, National Institute of Neurological Disorders and Stroke, National Institutes of Health, Bethesda, Maryland

Hemant S. Kelkar, Ph.D.
Postdoctoral Fellow, Texas A&M University, Department of Plantology and Microbiology, College Station, Texas

Darrell G. Kirch, M.D.
Dean, Schools of Medicine and Graduate Studies, Medical College of Georgia, Augusta, Georgia

William B. Lawson, M.D., Ph.D.
Associate Professor of Psychiatry, University of Arkansas for Medical Sciences, and Chief, Chronically Mentally Ill Section, Department of Psychiatry Services, North Little Rock VA Hospital, North Little Rock, Arkansas

Robert A. Leadbetter, M.D.
Clinical Associate Professor, Psychiatric Medicine, University of Virginia, and Director , Clinical Studies Unit, Western State Hospital, Staunton, Virginia

Daniel J. Luchins, M.D.
Associate Professor and Chief of Extramural Psychiatry, Department of Psychiatry, University of Chicago, Chicago, Illinois

Sahebarao P. Mahadik, Ph.D.
Professor, Department of Psychiatry and Health Behavior, Medical College of Georgia, Augusta, Georgia

Sukdeb Mukherjee, M.D. (Deceased)
Professor, Department of Psychiatry and Health Behavior, Medical College of Georgia, Augusta, Georgia

Diane Pavalonis, M.S.N., M.B.A.
Nurse Coordinator, Western State Hospital, Staunton, Virginia

David B. Schnur, M.D.
Assistant Professor of Psychiatry, Mt. Sinai School of Medicine, New York, New York, and Chief, Clinical Research Unit, Department of Psychiatry, Mt. Sinai Services, Elmhurst Hospital Center, Elmhurst, New York

Michael S. Shutty, Jr., Ph.D.
Clinical Assistant Professor of Anesthesiology, University of Virginia, and Clinical Psychologist, Western State Hospital, Staunton, Virginia

Scott Smith, M.A.
Clinical Research Unit, Mt. Sinai Services, Department of Psychiatry, Elmhurst Hospital Center, Elmhurst, New York

W. Victor R. Vieweg, M.D., F.A.C.P., F.A.C.C.
Professor of Psychiatry and Medicine, and Director of Geriatric Psychiatry, Department of Psychiatry, Medical College of Virginia, Virginia Commonwealth University, Richmond, Virginia

Introduction to the Progress in Psychiatry Series

The Progress in Psychiatry Series is designed to capture in print the excitement that comes from assembling a diverse group of experts from various locations to examine in detail the newest information about a developing aspect of psychiatry. This series emerged as a collaboration between the American Psychiatric Association's Scientific Program Committee and the American Psychiatric Press, Inc. Great interest is generated by a number of the symposia presented each year at the American Psychiatric Association annual meeting, and we realized that much of the information presented there, carefully assembled by people who are deeply immersed in a given area, would unfortunately not appear together in print. The symposia sessions at the annual meetings provide an unusual opportunity for experts who otherwise might not meet on the same platform to share their diverse viewpoints for 3 hours. Some new themes are repeatedly reinforced and gain credence, whereas in other instances disagreements emerge, enabling the audience and now the reader to reach informed decisions about new directions in the field. The Progress in Psychiatry Series allows us to publish and capture some of the best of the symposia and thus provide an in-depth treatment of specific areas that might not otherwise be presented in broader review formats.

Psychiatry is, by nature, an interface discipline, combining the study of mind and brain, of individual and social environments, of the humane and the scientific. Therefore, progress in the field is rarely linear—it often comes from unexpected sources. Furthermore, new developments emerge from an array of viewpoints that do not necessarily provide immediate agreement but rather expert examination of the issues. We intend to present innovative ideas and data that will enable you, the reader, to participate in this process.

We believe the Progress in Psychiatry Series will provide you with an opportunity to review timely information in specific fields of interest as they are developing. We hope you find that the excitement of the presentations is captured in the written word and that this book proves to be informative and enjoyable reading.

David Spiegel, M.D.
Series Editor
Progress in Psychiatry Series

Progress in Psychiatry
Series Titles

Water Balance in Schizophrenia (#48)
Edited by David B. Schnur, M.D., and Darrell G. Kirch, M.D.

NMR Spectroscopy in Psychiatric Brain Disorders (#47)
Edited by Henry A. Nasrallah, M.D., and Jay W. Pettegrew, M.D.

Does Stress Cause Psychiatric Illness? (#46)
Edited by Carolyn M. Mazure, Ph.D.

Biological and Neurobehavioral Studies of Borderline Personality Disorder (#45)
Edited by Kenneth R. Silk, M.D.

Severe Depressive Disorders (#44)
Edited by Leon Grunhaus, M.D., and John F. Greden, M.D.

Clinical Advances in Monoamine Oxidase Inhibitor Therapies (#43)
Edited by Sidney H. Kennedy, M.D., F.R.C.P.C.

Catecholamine Function in Posttraumatic Stress Disorder: Emerging Concepts (#42)
Edited by M. Michele Murburg, M.D.

Management and Treatment of Insanity Acquittees: A Model for the 1990s (#41)
Edited by Joseph D. Bloom, M.D., and Mary H. Williams, M.S., J.D.

Chronic Fatigue and Related Immune Deficiency Syndromes (#40)
Edited by Paul J. Goodnick, M.D., and Nancy G. Klimas, M.D.

Psychopharmacology and Psychobiology of Ethnicity (#39)
Edited by Keh-Ming Lin, M.D., M.P.H., Russell E. Poland, Ph.D.,
and Gayle Nakasaki, M.S.W.

**Electroconvulsive Therapy: From Research to Clinical
Practice (#38)**
Edited by C. Edward Coffey, M.D.

Multiple Sclerosis: A Neuropsychiatric Disorder (#37)
Edited by Uriel Halbreich, M.D.

Biology of Anxiety Disorders (#36)
Edited by Rudolf Hoehn-Saric, M.D., and Daniel R. McLeod, Ph.D.

Psychoimmunology Update (#35)
Edited by Jack M. Gorman, M.D., and Robert M. Kertzner, M.D.

Brain Imaging in Affective Disorders (#34)
Edited by Peter Hauser, M.D.

Positron-Emission Tomography in Schizophrenia Research (#33)
Edited by Nora D. Volkow, M.D., and Alfred P. Wolf, Ph.D.

Mental Retardation: Developing Pharmacotherapies (#32)
Edited by John J. Ratey, M.D.

**Current Concepts of Somatization: Research and Clinical
Perspectives (#31)**
Edited by Laurence J. Kirmayer, M.D., F.R.C.P.C., and James M.
Robbins, Ph.D.

**Central Nervous System Peptide Mechanisms in Stress and
Depression (#30)**
Edited by S. Craig Risch, M.D.

Neuropeptides and Psychiatric Disorders (#29)
Edited by Charles B. Nemeroff, M.D., Ph.D.

**Negative Schizophrenic Symptoms: Pathophysiology and
Clinical Implications (#28)**
Edited by John F. Greden, M.D., and Rajiv Tandon, M.D.

The Neuroleptic Nonresponsive Patient: Characterization and Treatment (#27)
Edited by Burt Angrist, M.D., and S. Charles Schulz, M.D.

Combination Pharmacotherapy and Psychotherapy for Depression (#26)
Edited by Donna Manning, M.D., and Allen J. Frances, M.D.

Treatment Strategies for Refractory Depression (#25)
Edited by Steven P. Roose, M.D., and Alexander H. Glassman, M.D.

Biological Rhythms, Mood Disorders, Light Therapy, and the Pineal Gland (#24)
Edited by Mohammad Shafii, M.D., and Sharon Lee Shafii, R.N., B.S.N.

Family Environment and Borderline Personality Disorder (#23)
Edited by Paul Skevington Links, M.D.

Amino Acids in Psychiatric Disease (#22)
Edited by Mary Ann Richardson, Ph.D.

Serotonin in Major Psychiatric Disorders (#21)
Edited by Emil F. Coccaro, M.D., and Dennis L. Murphy, M.D.

Personality Disorders: New Perspectives on Diagnostic Validity (#20)
Edited by John M. Oldham, M.D.

Biological Assessment and Treatment of Posttraumatic Stress Disorder (#19)
Edited by Earl L. Giller, Jr., M.D., Ph.D.

Depression in Schizophrenia (#18)
Edited by Lynn E. DeLisi, M.D.

Depression and Families: Impact and Treatment (#17)
Edited by Gabor I. Keitner, M.D.

Treatment of Affective Disorders in the Elderly (#3)
Edited by Charles A. Shamoian, M.D.

Premenstrual Syndrome: Current Findings and Future Directions (#2)
Edited by Howard J. Osofsky, M.D., Ph.D., and Susan J. Blumenthal, M.D.

The Borderline: Current Empirical Research (#1)
Edited by Thomas H. McGlashan, M.D.

Introduction

David B. Schnur, M.D.
Darrell G. Kirch, M.D.

The association between disturbances in water balance and schizophrenia has been recognized for more than half a century. Although initially thought to represent a benign condition, polydipsia and water imbalance were soon recognized as often causing water intoxication, in severe cases leading to delirium, coma, seizures, and even death. Since then, a great deal of research has been focused on various aspects of water dysregulation in patients with chronic psychosis. These efforts have been directed toward elucidating the pathophysiology, phenomenology, and treatment of polydipsia–hyponatremia syndrome. Our present aim has been to bring this research together in a single comprehensive volume on water balance and schizophrenia.

In this volume, the term *polydipsia–hyponatremia syndrome* is used to refer to a state of self-induced dilutional hyponatremia associated with the excessive drinking of fluids. *Water intoxication* denotes the changes in mental and neurological status that result from reductions in serum sodium and osmolality.

In the broadest sense of the term, *disordered water homeostasis* may be thought to comprise disturbances in the intake and excretion of water. When water balance was first evaluated in samples of chronically hospitalized psychiatric patients more than 60 years ago, abnormalities were found in a significant number of patients with schizophrenia and other diagnoses. More recently, when excessive diurnal weight gain was measured as an index of impaired water excretion, the majority of a sample of chronically institutionalized patients with schizophrenia was found to have abnormal diurnal weight increases reflecting disordered water balance. Moreover, it has been reported that water intoxication may be a leading cause of death in nongeriatric patients with chronic schizophrenia. Chapters

1 and 2 by Vieweg provide a history and review of many of the major research efforts pertinent to water dysregulation in schizophrenia and highlight the relatively high prevalence of the problem as well as the significant associated morbidity and mortality. Particular emphasis is placed on the interrelationship between polydipsia-hyponatremia syndrome seen in schizophrenia and other forms of water dysregulation, specifically those involving abnormalities in the hypothalamic-pituitary axis. It is noted that for water intoxication to occur, a disturbance in free water clearance must accompany polydipsia, pointing to possible dysregulation involving antidiuretic hormone. These observations have important implications for the prevention and treatment of water intoxication, because they provide a rationale for evaluating daily water intake by obtaining diurnal weights and point toward therapeutic strategies aimed at modifying the actions of antidiuretic hormone.

Investigators have just begun to focus on the physiological determinants of normal drinking behavior in the study of polydipsia-hyponatremia syndrome in schizophrenia. This research likely will enhance our understanding of the biology of polydipsia-hyponatremia syndrome and may lead to more effective treatment strategies.

In Chapter 3, Grossman describes the neuroanatomical structures subserving the regulation of thirst and clarifies the distinction between "intracellular" and "extracellular" thirst. The former is associated with increases in serum osmolality, whereas the latter results from hypovolemia. Recent findings suggest that dysregulation of intracellular thirst may subserve the polydipsia of chronic psychiatric patients. Chapter 3 also reviews the neuroendocrine regulation of thirst and the neuropharmacology of brain mechanisms that determine drinking behavior.

An understanding of the pathophysiology of water dysregulation in schizophrenia requires familiarity with cellular mechanisms of water homeostasis, a subject addressed by Mahadik, Mukherjee, and Kelkar in Chapter 4. The distribution of water within the body's intracellular and extracellular compartments is tightly regulated by the Na^+-K^+ pump, which, in turn, is dependent on the structural integrity of the cell membrane. The importance of the cell membrane in osmotic equilibrium is implied by evidence that disturbances in fatty acid distribution are associated with polydipsia in animals. The authors suggest that additional study of the relationship between membrane abnormalities and polydipsia will provide further insight into the physiological mechanisms regulating drinking behavior.

A number of investigators are applying our growing understanding of the normal physiological determinants of thirst, drinking, and water balance to studies of the ways in which these mechanisms might be disrupted in schizophrenia. An example of this research is the analysis of the regulation of antidiuretic hormone in schizophrenia. In Chapter 5, Goldman reviews evidence underscoring the importance of antidiuretic hormone dysregulation in polydipsia-hyponatremia syndrome. It is suggested that in this condition the osmotic threshold for antidiuretic hormone secretion and the slope of the antidiuretic hormone response to osmotic stimulation are both lowered. These alterations represent an enhanced response of antidiuretic hormone to increases in serum solutes and may underly chronic hyponatremia. However, such disturbances in antidiuretic hormone regulation are of insufficient magnitude to account for water intoxication. Thus, additional mechanisms that predominate during psychotic exacerbations and are associated with disturbances in limbic circuitry may be implicated.

A possible role for temporal lobe and limbic pathology in polydipsia-hyponatremia syndrome is suggested by diverse considerations. First, as reviewed by Elkashef, Leadbetter, and Kirch in Chapter 6, evidence from magnetic resonance imaging studies indicates that the amygdala–hippocampus is smaller in schizophrenia patients with polydipsia-hyponatremia syndrome compared with schizophrenia patients with normal water balance. Preliminary data suggest that this finding is not a transitory consequence of the acute intake of large amounts of fluid but rather represents a primary alteration in brain morphology. Second, animal studies described in Chapter 7 by Luchins and Canuso indicate that hippocampal damage may result in polydipsia, particularly under conditions of fixed schedule food reinforcement. These authors review the role of temporal lobe disturbances in the pathophysiology of schizophrenia and argue that a variety of manneristic behaviors including polydipsia may involve hippocampal dysfunction. Finally, the cognitive impairments associated with polydipsia-hyponatremia syndrome are described in Chapter 8 by Schnur and Smith, who suggest that these may originate from temporal lobe disturbances.

In a somewhat different vein, Mahadik and colleagues, in Chapter 4, suggest that abnormalities in cell membrane structure hypothesized to subserve polydipsia-hyponatremia syndrome may overlap with those reported in the general population of patients with schizophrenia. The implication is that much may be learned about the pathophysiology of schizophrenia by studying the determinants of polydipsia-hyponatremia syndrome. This idea is consistent with the view that the structural brain pathology observed by Elkashef and colleagues (Chapter 6) using magnetic resonance imaging in patients with polydipsia-hyponatremia syndrome is simply a greater degree of the structural abnormalities observed in schizophrenia in general. Similarly, Schnur and Smith (Chapter 8) suggest that polydipsia-hyponatremia syndrome may represent a characteristic of the schizophrenic defect state and as such provide insights into the pathophysiology of schizophrenia.

Regardless of its role in our understanding of schizophrenia, polydipsia is easily reproduced in animals, suggesting that experimental manipulations that alter drinking behavior in animals may provide information on the pathophysiology of polydipsia-hyponatremia syndrome in schizophrenia and other chronic psychiatric disorders. This evidence is considered by a number of the authors (Chapters 1–5).

The management of polydipsia-hyponatremia syndrome and its complications presents a particular challenge to the clinician because it requires familiarity with both the behavioral and the medical aspects of this condition. A precipitous drop in serum concentration may result in water intoxication, a medical emergency requiring immediate intervention. As indicated by Karp (Chapter 9), the most serious insult to the brain's structural integrity supervenes when a sudden drop in plasma osmolality is so great that compensatory mechanisms are overwhelmed. The result is cerebral edema and the ensuing clinical manifestations of water intoxication. Therapeutic strategies aim at reestablishing normal plasma osmolality but must take into account the danger of inducing central pontine myelinolysis. The risks of hyponatremia must be weighed against those associated with excessively rapid correction of hyponatremia. After reviewing the pertinent literature, Karp provides recommendations for the treatment of acute water intoxication.

Vigilant day-to-day management of patients with polydipsia-hyponatremia syndrome is critical in preventing water intoxication. The major aim of treatment is to intervene before the patient has consumed dangerous quantities of fluids. Achieving this goal using traditional methods of care is staff intensive, because it often requires one-to-one monitoring of the patient's fluid restriction regimen. An alternate approach, described by Leadbetter, Shutty, Hammersberg, Higgens, and Pavalonis in Chapter 10, makes use of a therapeutic inpatient unit specializing in the treatment of polydipsia-hyponatremia syndrome. These authors provide a comprehensive review of the inpatient assessment and treatment of abnormal drinking behavior. They emphasize that behavioral as well as pharmacological therapeutic techniques are indicated and that management must involve family members. Although a "water drinkers ward" does not provide a definitive solution for the problem of polydipsia-hyponatremia syndrome, it represents a less-restrictive means of ensuring patient safety and may improve quality of life.

Despite recent advances in our understanding of the pathophysiology of polydipsia-hyponatremia syndrome, specific pharmacological treatments for this condition have not been developed. Perhaps the most promising agent is clozapine, but its efficacy in preventing water intoxication has not yet been supported by systematic studies. In Chapter 11, Lawson reviews the extensive array of medications that have been proposed as treatments for polydipsia-hyponatremia syndrome and concludes that further study is needed to provide definitive information on efficacy. At present several available agents act on a variety of physiological mechanisms thought to be disturbed in polydipsia-hyponatremia syndrome. Although many of these drugs have been reported to be beneficial in specific instances, a critical perusal of the literature suggests that such claims are at best tentative.

To our knowledge this volume represents the first attempt to consolidate the diverse areas of research focused on polydipsia-hyponatremia syndrome associated with schizophrenia. Where possible, attempts have been made to provide details regarding methodology and explicit guidelines in management. However, the reader immediately will become aware that the questions asked in this volume are more numerous than the answers provided. It is hoped that these questions will define the limitations of our current knowledge and serve as a springboard for future study.

Chapter 1

Overview

W. Victor R. Vieweg, M.D., F.A.C.P., F.A.C.C.

EARLY HISTORY

Polydipsia and Polyuria

Early research on polydipsia attempted to shed light on mechanisms subserving diabetes insipidus. In 1905, Schäfer and Herring studied the renal diuretic action of pituitary extracts. After injecting saline extracts of the pituitary body infundibulum into *anesthetized* dogs, these workers observed blood pressure and urine flow changes. Because they noted increased urine flow, they concluded that pituitary extract was a diuretic. They believed that diabetes insipidus resulted from posterior pituitary lobe overactivity. This assertion confused distinctions between primary polydipsia and diabetes insipidus (Achard and Ramond 1905; Ebstein 1909; Reichardt 1908).

Independently, von den Velden (1913) in Germany and Farini and Ceccaroni (1913) in Italy administered pituitary extract to *unanesthetized* patients with diabetes insipidus. This administration relieved thirst, polydipsia, and polyuria. Both teams concluded that diabetes insipidus derived from posterior pituitary lobe underactivity. Schäfer and Herring (1905) failed to appreciate that anesthetizing their dogs confounded assessing pituitary posterior lobe function. If their saline extracts of the pituitary body infundibulum were contaminated with prolactin from the anterior lobe, prolactin may have induced diuresis (R. A. Adler et al. 1986).

Water Intoxication

Between 1921 and 1923, Rowntree and colleagues (Rowntree 1922, 1923; Weir et al. 1922) studied diabetes insipidus and water balance. Investigations of water-loaded animals led to the idea of water intoxication. These systematic studies, controlling the pace and sequence of symptoms and signs of water intoxication, continue to shape our understanding of dilutional hyponatremia among patients with chronic schizophrenia.

After talking to patients with diabetes insipidus, Rowntree and colleagues (Rowntree 1923; Weir et al. 1922) concluded that thirst and polydipsia preceded polyuria in this entity. (We now know that polyuria precedes polydipsia in diabetes insipidus, and polydipsia precedes polyuria in the polydipsia-hyponatremia syndrome.) Their patients excreted 3–14 L per day and had urine specific gravities of 1.001–1.004. Administering pituitary extract reversed these abnormal findings. The investigators asked one patient with diabetes insipidus to continue drinking his usual amount of water after taking pituitary extract. He ingested 5.25 L of water and excreted 800 ml of urine over the next 8 hours (Weir et al. 1922). He developed nausea, headache, and lower eyelid and ankle edema. Other patients who continued to drink water after taking pituitary extract experienced nausea, vomiting, headache, ataxia, and the need to lie down.

Stimulated by these clinical observations in humans, the authors gave large quantities of water to dogs after administering pituitary extract subcutaneously. In early experiments, Weir et al. (1922) gave dogs 50 ml of water per kilogram of body weight each hour via a gastric tube. (This is the equivalent of 84 L per day in a 70-kg human.) Early manifestations of water intoxication included weakness, restlessness, polyuria, diarrhea, and vomiting. Tremor and salivation followed these features. The animals became drowsy, showed muscle twitching, and became ataxic. Weir et al. (1922) called this the preconvulsive stage. Later manifestations of water intoxication (called the convulsive stage) included tonic then clonic seizures, coma, and death. The authors showed that neither water intake (at a rate of 50 ml/hour) nor pituitary extract alone produced this sequence of events. They postulated that pituitary extract facilitated water intoxication either by reducing urine formation and excretion or by promoting intravascular water transfer into extravascular tissues.

In a second set of experiments, Rowntree (1923) gave water more rapidly and without supplemental pituitary extract. Every 30 minutes, animals (dogs, cats, rabbits, and guinea pigs) took 50 ml of water per kilogram of body weight via a gastric tube. (This is the equivalent of 168 L per day for a 70-kg human.) Along with the clinical features previously mentioned, the authors reported marked bradycardia with severe water intoxication. (This may be another mechanism contributing to sudden death in the polydipsia-hyponatremia syndrome.) During these experiments, the range of animal weight gain at death, as a fraction of initial weight, was 8.0%–26.3% for rabbits, 9.7%–52.2% for guinea pigs, and 12.0%–50.0% for cats. (For a 70-kg human using these percentages corresponding to the range of weight gains from onset of water loading until death would be 5.6–18.4 kg, 6.8–36.8 kg, and 8.4–35.0 kg, respectively.)

Rowntree (1923) developed the concept of subacute water intoxication (contrasted with the earlier studies of acute water intoxication). He noted that rabbits could tolerate daily water intake (without coadministration of pituitary extract) equaling up to one-fourth of body weight for 2–3 weeks without developing water intoxication. When these investigators gave from 300 to 333 ml of water per kilogram of body weight each day, the syndrome of subacute water intoxication developed. (For a 70-kg human, comparable daily water intake would range from 21 to 23.3 L.) As in acute water intoxication, features of subacute water intoxication included salivation, listlessness, ataxia, polyuria, fright, and disinterest. Later, weakness and stupor occurred followed by seizures, coma, and death. Experiments with dogs showed that increased intracranial pressure and autopsy findings of cerebral edema accompanied water intoxication. Subacute rather than acute water intoxication in animals is probably more similar to the water intoxication found in schizophrenic patients with the polydipsia-hyponatremia syndrome.

Rowntree (1923) documented the efficacy of intravenous administration of hypertonic (10% sodium chloride) saline in water intoxication. Dogs in stupor, seizures, or coma recovered within 15–30 minutes of treatment.

Editorial review (Editor 1953) of Rowntree's work criticized applying the term "water intoxication" to his clinical observations. The editor suggested that this term delayed recognizing the seriousness of this syndrome, because everyone *knows* that it is safe to drink water and that we cannot voluntarily drink too much water. The editor argued that it is not the absolute excess of total body water but the water-to-electrolyte ratio, particularly hypotonic extracellular solutions, that drives water into cells and leads to water intoxication. Whereas the editor did not use the term "dilutional hyponatremia," he argued that such a term is preferred to the term "water intoxication." Because laboratories did not commonly measure serum sodium concentration until the 1940s, we can forgive Rowntree's focus on water toxicity rather than water-sodium mismatch.

Polydipsia, Schizophrenia, and Water Intoxication

Between 1928 and 1933, Hoskins and colleagues (Hoskins 1933; Hoskins and Sleeper 1933; Sleeper 1935; Sleeper and Jellinek 1936) used a 7-month protocol to study various clinical and laboratory parameters among 300 patients with schizophrenia at Worcester State Hospital. Among 44 schizophrenic men (Hoskins 1933), daily urine volume was 2602 ± 1851 ml (range 510–8,000 ml) compared with 26 control-group males' value of 1,328 ± 629 ml (range 655–2,805 ml). The investigators catheterized patients to obtain daily urine volumes. Converting from urine creatinine nitrogen content, the daily urine creatinine concentration was 49.55 ± 33.88 mg/dl or 19.7 mg per kilogram of body weight for 57 male patients (Hoskins and Sleeper 1933). Serum sodium concentration was not measured.

Hoskins' group (Sleeper 1935) showed that polyuric schizophrenic patients excreted similar urine volumes each day. For two adjacent 24-hour urine volumes, the intraclass correlation was 0.78 ± 0.04. Over the 7-month study, during which time they collected six daily urine volumes, the intraclass correlation was 0.70. The investigators recommended catheterizing patients to avoid residual urine volume confounding urine volume measurement.

Hoskins (1933) concluded that hypothalamic or posterior pituitary lobe dysfunction explained these findings and that the polyuria of schizophrenia was benign. They may have eliminated patients from their study with greater degrees of polyuria and episodes of water intoxication. Whereas Hoskins' group knew that patients with psychiatric disorders occasionally suffered from polydipsia and polyuria and that such polydipsia was often called primary, hysterical, or psychogenic polydipsia, they were surprised to find that polyuria was a common feature of chronic schizophrenia.

Helwig et al. (1935) first reported a human fatality from water intoxication. A 50-year-old woman underwent cholecystectomy without incident. She received 9,000 ml of tap water administered by proctoclysis (rectal tube) over the 30-hour period following surgery. Postoperative symptoms and signs included neck pain, perspiration, vomiting, severe headache, tremor, stupor, seizures, coma, and death 41 hours after surgery. The authors performed an autopsy within 1 hour of death (before either rigor mortis or livor mortis appeared). Findings included extensive cerebral edema. Helwig et al. (1935) then induced water intoxication in seven rabbits by giving 50 ml of tap water rectally every 30 minutes. They noted a decrease in serum chloride concentration (they did not measure serum sodium concentration) and extensive visceral and cerebral edema at autopsy consistent with those of their deceased patient findings and with the findings of Rowntree and his group (Rowntree 1923; Weir et al. 1922).

Water intoxication was first described in a schizophrenic patient in 1938 (Barahal 1938). After a generalized seizure, a 31-year-old woman with paranoid schizophrenia and polydipsia vomited a large amount of water. Facial edema was present. She had several more seizures over the next 7 hours and vomited more water. She remained drowsy for 5 days. Although he did not measure serum chloride concentration, Barahal (1938) concluded that the patient experienced water intoxication.

Idiopathic Polydipsia Versus Diabetes Insipidus

Increased fluid ingestion occurs in both idiopathic polydipsia and diabetes insipidus. Because both entities have different pathophysiological determinants and different treatments, distinguishing between them is important.

Initial attempts to distinguish between idiopathic polydipsia and diabetes insipidus was based on clinical observation (Bauer 1925). However, by the 1940s, Hickey and Hare (1944) had developed a procedure using intravenous hypertonic saline to make this distinction more precisely. After hypertonic saline stimulation, the investigators collected the urine and recovered the antidiuretic substance, pituitrin, by dialysis. Then, dogs with surgically induced diabetes insipidus received the substance intravenously. They retained fluid with coadministration of as little as 0.1 mU of pituitrin. This procedure was a primitive biological assay for antidiuretic hormone.

Subsequently, Hickey and Hare (1944) adapted this procedure for humans as follows. The healthy or polyuric subject drank 20 ml of water per kilogram of body weight in less than 1 hour. Then for 45 minutes, the subject received 2.5% sodium chloride intravenously at a rate of 0.25 ml per kilogram of body weight. Measured urine collections (preferably obtained by catheterization) at 15-minute intervals before, during, and after saline injection distinguished between idiopathic polydipsia and diabetes insipidus. Water loading produced a diuresis that was reversed (an antidiuretic state was induced) with hypertonic saline challenge in subjects with an intact pituitary gland posterior lobe. In subjects with diabetes insipidus, antidiuresis did not take place.

Water restriction also may be used to distinguish between diabetes insipidus and idiopathic polydipsia. For example, Díes et al. (1961) argued that intravenous administration of vasopressin immediately after dehydration could best distinguish between idiopathic polydipsia and diabetes insipidus. They diagnosed diabetes insipidus if vasopressin administration produced a more concentrated urine than did dehydration; if not, the authors diagnosed idiopathic polydipsia.

Similarly, Dashe et al. (1963) used a standardized 6.5-hour water deprivation test in the differential diagnosis of polyuria. They found that polyuric subjects had initial serum osmolality determinations ranging from 273 to 293 mOsm/kg, had remarkable consistency of serum osmolality measurements throughout the water deprivation test, and had a urine-to-serum osmolality ratio of ≥ 100.9. Patients with diabetes insipidus were unable to concentrate their urine fully. Those subjects needing vasopressin replacement had serum osmolality concentrations ≥ 300 mOsm/kg. By contrast, individuals with primary polydipsia had stable serum osmolality determinations at normal or slightly less than normal levels and normal urine osmolality measurements at the end of testing. In an illuminating case study, Fricchoine et al. (1987) described concomitant diabetes insipidus and idiopathic polydipsia in a 42-year-old woman with chronic schizophrenia. Admission serum sodium concentration was 175 mmol/L, plasma osmolality was 359 mOsm/kg, urine osmolality was 392 mOsm/kg, and renal function was normal without glycosuria. Findings thought consistent with diabetes insipidus included 1) water deprivation testing with baseline urine osmolality 66 mOsm/kg and 6-hour value 358 mOsm/kg and 2) later vasopressin challenge (intranasal desmopressin acetate [DDAVP] every 12 hours) and fluid challenge (> 6 L of water per day) causing serum sodium concentration to decrease to 120 mmol/L. After stabilization, serum sodium concentration ranged from 132 to 145 mmol/L, and the patient drank water freely (6–8 L per day). The authors gave haloperidol as the only drug. The disassociation between thirst and osmotic regulation was proposed to explain the finding that vasopressin concentrations were low or absent at the same time that the thirst drive was unusually active in the same patient. The authors concluded that distinguishing between idiopathic polydipsia and central diabetes insipidus may be impossible at times.

Compulsive Water Drinking

Barlow and De Wardener (1959) studied patterns of polydipsia among seven women and two men. Although the authors used the term "compulsive water drinkers" to describe their patients, we would now consider them as having the polydipsia-hyponatremia syndrome. Neurotic and dramatic traits, affective lability, history of vague illness during childhood, sleep walking, and sex life dissatisfaction and instability were common features of the study population. A few patients smoked.

History of polydipsia ranged from 4 months to 20 years, and its onset was usually insidious. Disturbances included severe delusions, depression, agitation, indifference, tunnel vision, and facial mannerisms. Daily urine volumes ranged between 2.5 and 5 L for the least polydipsic subject and between 13 and 20 L for the most polydipsic subject. (Normal values for daily urine volume are up to 2,600 ml for men and up to 2,200 ml for women weighing 70 and 60 kg, respectively. This is equivalent to 37 ml/kg of body weight for both sexes [Vieweg et al. 1988i].) The mean plasma osmolality was lower for patients (269 mOsm/kg) than for control subjects (280 mOsm/kg).

When given intravenous vasopressin, urine concentrating ability was lower in patients than in control subjects. During fluid deprivation, control subjects concentrated their urine more than patients. When given long-acting vasopressin, patients continued to drink water and experienced headache, nausea, vomiting, abdominal distension, skin tightening, anger, and dissociation. Polydipsia without supplemental vasopressin did not lead to symptomatic dilutional hyponatremia.

Barlow and De Wardener (1959) found that basal plasma osmolality was greatest for patients with diabetes insipidus and least for compulsive water drinkers with control subjects between these two groups. When given long-acting vasopressin, diabetes insipidus patients lost their thirst and compulsive water drinkers remained thirsty. Narcotherapy in two and electroconvulsive treatments in another two compulsive water drinkers temporarily reduced polydipsia.

Adding patients from the literature to their own subjects, Barlow and De Wardener (1959) reported that 79% of 19 compulsive water drinkers were women. The age of onset of polydipsia was 8–18 years in four patients, 35–59 years in 14 patients, and uncertain in one patient. Among subjects with diabetes insipidus, 41% were women. Diabetes insipidus developed most commonly before age 20 years. Barlow and De Wardener's article supports the misperception that the polydipsia-hyponatremia syndrome is more common among women than men.

THIRST

Early Studies

The work by Cannon (1919) on the origins of thirst dominated the thinking on this subject during the first half of the 20th century. He proposed that the "water supply is maintained because we avoid, or abolish, by taking water or aqueous fluid, the disagreeable sensations that arise and torment us with increasing torment if the salivary glands, because of a lowering of the water-content of the body, lack the water they need to function, and fail therefore to pour out their watery secretion in sufficient amount and in proper quality to keep moist the mouth and pharynx" (p. 301). This theory of the local origin of thirst was analogous to his theory that the sensation of hunger derived from contractions of the stomach.

Disorders of Thirst

Anticipated and habitual drinking, as opposed to thirst-motivated behavior, usually satisfies our need for water. We have, however, an efficient thirst mechanism and appropriate regulation of arginine vasopressin secretion to maintain optimal water balance under water-deficit conditions. Altered fluid balance that elicits thirst also stimulates vasopressin release from the posterior lobe of the pituitary gland. It appears that vasopressin secretion and water intake are regulated by essentially identical enteroceptor mechanisms in the supraoptic and paraventricular nuclei of the hypothalamus (Andersson and Rundgren 1982). The enteroceptor mechanisms have a lower stimulus threshold to stimulate osmotic vasopressin release than to elicit thirst; a 1%–2% change in osmolality alters vasopressin release, whereas thirst is stimulated at a threshold of about a 2% deficit in total body water (Robertson et al. 1976). The order of priorities that stimulate vasopressin release and thirst are 1) water loss without corresponding sodium loss (hypertonic dehydration) and 2) an osmotic shift of intracellular water to extracellular water resulting from excessive salt intake. Although there is no net loss of water in the latter condition, both conditions represent cellular dehydration, hyperosmolality of the body fluids, and elevated extracellular sodium concentration. Of these three factors, it is believed that cellular dehydration drives both vasopressin release and thirst. This kind of regulation is designated osmotic following the work of Verney (1947) showing that vasopressin release correlates inversely with the volume of cerebral osmoreceptors. We still do not know whether volume change or sodium concentration change drives these sensory mechanisms.

Volume regulation usually parallels and complements osmotic regulation. In humans, about a 10% reduction in blood volume must occur before plasma vasopressin increases (Robertson and Athar 1976). When, however, a discordant volume–osmotic signal is sent to the hypothalamus to govern vasopressin secretion, the volume signal overrides the osmotic signal. For example, making animals hypotonic signals the hypothalamus to prevent vasopressin release. Then if such animals are suddenly bled to a hypovolemic state, a new signal is sent to the hypothalamus to secrete vasopressin to preserve body water in preference to preserving electrolyte balance.

Normally, osmoregulatory thirst appears to be an emergency mechanism that operates only when water in food and anticipated or habitual drinking combined with maximal vasopressin effect fail to maintain extracellular sodium concentration below a certain set point. This regulatory pattern is congruent with the observation that hypothalamic enteroceptor mechanisms have a lower stimulus threshold to stimulate osmotic vasopressin release than to elicit thirst (Andersson and Rundgren 1982) and would lead to the prediction that dilutional hyponatremia would precede thirst dysregulation in schizophrenia. Paradoxically, however, polydipsia precedes hyponatremia by more than a decade in schizophrenia (Vieweg et al. 1984d). An explanation for this relationship may involve altered patterns of anticipation and habit. Alternatively, schizophrenia-induced neurodevelopmental or neurodegenerative changes in the paraventricular and supraoptic nuclei of the hypothalamus may explain the polydipsia-hyponatremia progression paradox in schizophrenia. A third possibility is that subtle changes in osmotic regulation occur early in schizophrenia but are not manifest clinically until much later in the illness.

Thirst Satisfaction

Water must be absorbed in sufficient quantities to return cerebral sensors below levels required to stimulate the urge to drink before the animal stops water-seeking behavior. Satisfaction of thirst occurs at a higher threshold than the urge to drink, thereby providing a water reserve that can be lost before the urge to drink returns (Fitzsimons 1979). Without this mechanism, we would drink water excessively whenever we became thirsty and then have to endure profuse water diuresis. Disruption of this mechanism could explain polydipsia and polyuria in schizophrenia.

Snyder (1984) reported that opiate agonists bind up to 50 times more powerfully in hypotonic solutions compared with eutonic solutions. Opiate receptors highly concentrate in numerous structures of the limbic system, particularly the amygdala. Could patients with polydipsia-hyponatremia syndrome drink water (water "addiction") to dilute extracellular fluid so that opiate receptors bind more powerfully and give patients a "high?"

Dopamine, Vasopressin, and Thirst

Evidence from Lightman and Forsling (1980) suggests that dopamine may subserve vasopressin regulation at the level of the pituitary gland or the median eminence of the hypothalamus. These authors reported six normal young subjects (four men and two women, ages 20–22 years) randomly completing three protocols. In the control phase, subjects received sodium chloride intravenously as they moved from the supine to a head-up position on a tilt table. In the second experiment, subjects received L-dopa intravenously. Subjects took the decarboxilase inhibitor, carbidopa, 2 hours before receiving intravenous L-dopa in the third phase. Administration of L-dopa alone was associated with a significant drop in vasopressin in the supine position and an inhibition of the rise in vasopressin in response to tilt. However, such vasopressin inhibition was not observed with preadministration of carbidopa. It is known that carbidopa, which does not cross the blood-brain barrier, inhibits the decarboxilation of L-dopa to dopamine. Therefore, reversal of L-dopa inhibition of vasopressin by carbidopa preadministration was thought to implicate the pituitary or median eminence of the hypothalamus as possible sites of dopamine action as these are the only hypothalamo–hypophysial structures outside the blood-brain barrier. The authors found that when they gave L-dopa, there was a significant fall in vasopressin when subjects were supine and an inhibition in the rise of vasopressin in response to tilt. This effect is most likely mediated by L-dopa's metabolic product dopamine produced in brain tissue containing the enzyme dopa decarboxylase. When subjects took both carbidopa and L-dopa, they lost L-dopa's inhibition of vasopressin release. Because carbidopa does not cross the blood-brain barrier, its inhibition of the decarboxylation of L-dopa to dopamine must take place outside the blood-brain barrier. The pituitary gland and the median eminence of the hypothalamus are the only components of the hypothalamo–hypophysial system located outside the blood-brain barrier. It follows that the central nervous system conversion of L-dopa to dopamine (and by that, the inhibition of vasopressin release) takes place in the pituitary gland or the median eminence of the hypothalamus.

Shen and Sata (1983) suggested that water intoxication derives from hypothalamic dopaminergic supersensitivity, a mechanism analogous to striatal dopaminergic supersensitivity proposed to cause tardive dyskinesia. They studied chronically psychotic patients with polydipsia-hyponatremia syndrome. Six of 45 subjects developed water intoxication after their antipsychotic drug dose was reduced. Later, Shen and Sata (1984) asserted that antipsychotic drug-dose reduction may lead to increased thirst and vasopressin release via hypothalamic dopaminergic supersensitivity. Jones (1984) argued similarly, pointing out that dopamine controls both thirst and osmotic regulation and that haloperidol inhibits thirst when injected centrally. It follows that antipsychotic drug withdrawal may increase thirst and vasopressin release leading to water intoxication.

Work by R. A. Adler et al. (1986) showed that hyperprolactinemia in rats may induce diuresis and promote fluid ingestion. The animals had extra anterior pituitary glands implanted under the kidney capsule to induce endogenous hyperprolactinemia. When adjusted for fluid intake, endogenous hyperprolactinemia increased urine flow in rats. Extrapolating these animal findings to humans suggests that because of their prolactin-elevating effect, we must exclude antipsychotic drugs as the cause of polydipsia in polydipsia-hyponatremia syndrome.

However, when Vieweg et al. (1985b) decreased or eliminated antipsychotic drug dosage in patients with polydipsia–hyponatremia syndrome, there was worsening of polydipsia, hyponatremia, and psychosis. Increasing, not decreasing, antipsychotic drug dose among polydipsic-hyponatremic patients was the more promising course. On the other hand, in a second study, Vieweg et al. (1989b) found a weak, but statistically significant, correlation between antipsychotic drug dose and diurnal weight gain (and degree of dilutional hyponatremia) in patients with poly-dipsia-hyponatremia syndrome. This latter relationship does not necessarily imply that diurnal weight gain is the result of neuroleptic treatment. An equally plausible explanation is that patients with polydipsia-hyponatremia syndrome required high antipsychotic drug doses because of severity of illness (Vieweg et al. 1989f). In another study, Vieweg et al. (1989c) found no correlation between antipsychotic drug dose and diurnal weight gain in patients with polydipsia-hyponatremia syndrome. Whatever effect antipsychotic drugs may have on water balance in schizophrenia, polydipsia-hyponatremia syndrome long antedated the introduction of antipsychotic drugs, and the role of prolactin in water regulation in humans remains poorly defined.

ANTIDIURETIC HORMONE AND THE SYNDROME OF INAPPROPRIATE ANTIDIURESIS

Verney (1947) showed that injecting hypertonic saline into the carotid artery of conscious, hydrated dogs caused a fall in urine output similar to that found after pituitary extract administration. Solute concentration in the blood circulating in the supraopticohypophyseal system normally controls antidiuretic hormone secretion. Increased (hyperosmolar) solute concentration at this site stimulated release of antidiuretic hormone from the posterior pituitary lobe into the circulation. Decreased (hypoosmolar) solute concentration blocked antidiuretic hormone release. Verney also recognized that there were nonosmotic factors influencing antidiuretic hormone release, including intravascular volume and emotional stress.

The Syndrome of Inappropriate Antidiuresis

Schwartz et al. (1957) described two patients with bronchogenic carcinoma who had symptoms of hyponatremia, renal salt loss, and serum more hypotonic than urine. Both patients underwent extensive physiological evaluation before dying of cancer. The authors concluded that antidiuretic hormone was secreted inappropriately in both cases. Three years later, Schwartz et al. (1960) described a third patient with bronchogenic carcinoma and inappropriate antidiuretic hormone secretion. Continuing renal sodium loss distinguished this patient with dilutional hyponatremia from those with cardiac or hepatic failure.

Bartter and Schwartz (1967) described the pathophysiology, differential diagnosis, and treatment of patients with the syndrome of inappropriate antidiuresis. Clinical features included 1) hyponatremia and hypoosmolality of serum and extracellular fluid, 2) continued renal sodium loss, 3) no clinical findings of hypovolemia, 4) failure to maximally dilute the urine–urine osmolality greater than appropriate for the concomitant plasma tonicity, 5) normal renal function, and 6) normal adrenal function. If the serum sodium concentration was > 120 mmol/L, most patients were asymptomatic. When dilutional hyponatremia became more severe, patients lost their appetite; developed nausea and vomiting; and became irritable, uncooperative, and hostile. When serum sodium concentration dropped to < 110 mmol/L, neurological signs appeared including hyporeflexia, asthenia, bulbar or pseudobulbar palsy, positive Babinski's sign, stupor, and seizures. When serum sodium concentration was in the 90–105 mmol/L range, neurological consequences were severe and some patients died.

Polydipsic psychiatric patients may become hyponatremic without elevated levels of antidiuretic hormone, according to Bartter and Schwartz (1967), if fluid consumption exceeds renal excretion capacity. They asserted that renal water excretion cannot exceed 25 ml per minute based on the following assumptions and calculations. Urine dilution capacity (lowest urine osmolality level) and total solute available for excretion limit urine volume. If the lowest possible urine osmolality level is 50 mOsm/kg and the 24-hour solute load is 1,800 mOsm/kg, to be excreted in the urine, urine volume cannot exceed 25 ml per minute (25 ml per minute x 1,440 minutes per day = 36 L per day. 36 L per day x 50 mOsm/kg = 1,800 mOsm/kg per day).

Treatments for the syndrome of inappropriate antidiuresis available to Bartter and Schwartz (1967) included fluid restriction and hypertonic saline administration. They restricted fluid intake to 500–700 ml per day to achieve a total weight loss of 2–4 kg. They used hypertonic saline infusion when seizures or coma pointed to severe water intoxication.

Syndrome of Inappropriate Antidiuresis Versus the Syndrome of Inappropriate Antidiuretic Hormone

The "appropriateness" of antidiuretic hormone secretion relates to serum or plasma osmolality or sodium concentration (Schrier 1974). When serum sodium concentration is high, we expect "osmoreceptors" near the third ventricle or supraoptic or paraventricular nuclei of the hypothalamus (osmostat) to stimulate antidiuretic hormone release from the posterior pituitary lobe, thereby facilitating water reabsorption from the renal distal tubules and collecting ducts. If serum sodium concentration is low, we expect a reduction or extinction of antidiuretic hormone release to facilitate renal free water clearance and return serum sodium concentration to normal. Extracellular osmolality does not exclusively control physiological antidiuretic hormone secretion. Such nonosmotic factors as volume, pain, fear, and stress influence antidiuretic hormone levels. Hormone concentrations, therefore, may be very appropriate for the nonosmotic stimulus or stimuli, even though levels are discordant with serum sodium concentration. The syndrome of inappropriate antidiuresis is a more useful concept than the syndrome of inappropriate antidiuretic hormone. Antidiuresis poses the problem, not circulating antidiuretic hormone levels.

Arginine Vasopressin Measurements

In healthy control subjects with plasma osmolality greater than 280 mOsm/kg, plasma vasopressin increases linearly with increasing plasma tonicity (plasma vasopressin = 0.38 x [plasma osmolality in mOsm/kg – 280]). Below this plasma osmolality threshold, plasma vasopressin concentration falls to < 1 pg/ml (Robertson et al. 1976), permitting diuresis of at least 10–20 L per day. The hypo-thalamic osmostat regulates water balance within a plasma osmo-lality tolerance of < 1% (Weitzman and Kleeman 1979).

In patients meeting Bartter-Schwartz criteria (Bartter and Schwartz 1967) for the syndrome of inappropriate antidiuresis, Robertson and colleagues (Zerbe et al. 1980) studied 79 patients using a very sensi-tive radioimmunoassay for vasopressin measurement. In 80% of their patients, basal vasopressin measurements were comparable to val-ues found in normally hydrated healthy adults. However, the re-sponse to hypertonic saline infusion and/or water loading demonstrated four patterns of abnormal vasopressin secretion in patients with the syndrome of inappropriate antidiuresis. This tech-nology divided the study sample into four groups. In 37% of pa-tients (group 1), there was no relationship between plasma osmolality and vasopressin measurements. In group 2 (33% of patients), the osmotic threshold was abnormally low (reset osmostat), although the relationship between plasma osmolality and vasopressin was preserved. A nonsuppressible vasopressin leak was present in group 3 (16% of patients). Here, plasma vasopressin increased as plasma osmolality increased after hypertonic saline challenge. With water loading, vasopressin concentration did not fall when the plasma osmolality dropped below 278 mOsm/kg. In the last and smallest group (group 4, 14% of patients), vasopressin levels were unmeasurable after water loading among patients who could not maximally dilute their urine (hypovasopressinemic form). None of the four groups was associated with specific illnesses. A patient could change from one group to another group on repeat testing. Patients tended, however, to remain in the same group on retesting.

SCHIZOPHRENIA AND THE SYNDROME OF INAPPROPRIATE ANTIDIURESIS

Hobson and English (1963) reported the association of polydipsia, dilutional hyponatremia, the syndrome of inappropriate anti-diuresis, and schizophrenia. They described a 38-year-old man with alcoholism and schizophrenia who, when evaluated at the National Institute of Mental Health, had polydipsia and polyuria (mean daily urine volume 3,200 ml). In the hospital, he had a generalized seizure in the early afternoon. After the seizure was a brief period of lucidity followed by agitation, confusion, and urinary incontinence. Two hours after the seizure, serum sodium concentration was 109 mmol/L, urine specific gravity was 1.003, and blood urea nitrogen was 5 mg/dl. The patient received hypertonic saline and steroids. Twelve hours later, the serum osmolality was 262 mOsm/kg and the urine osmolality was 610 mOsm/kg. For the next 3 days, daily urine volume ranged from 800 to 1,200 ml, and serum sodium concentration ranged from 130 to 135 mmol/L.

After an overnight fast, the patient was water loaded (1,500 ml in 15 minutes). Although the patient's serum was hypotonic, he could not maximally dilute his urine consistent with the syndrome of inappropriate antidiuresis. The patient could conserve renal sodium when eating a 500-mg sodium diet and taking fluids ad libitum. While the patient was receiving a normal sodium diet, large amounts of sodium appeared in the urine. Case reports followed, documenting the association of psychosis and the syndrome of inappropriate antidiuresis (Dubovsky et al. 1973; Fowler et al. 1977; Inoue et al. 1985; Kramer and Drake 1983; Raskind et al. 1975; Rosenbaum et al. 1979; Vieweg et al. 1986e), although controversy continued about whether polydipsia alone could lead to water intoxication (W. O. Smith and Clark 1980).

Shortly after Hobson and English's report (1963), Mandell et al. (1964) related fluid retention to the degree of psychological disturbance. They measured free water clearance and anxiety in 10 patients and showed that decreased anxiety and increased free water clearance related positively.

Hariprasad et al. (1980) described 20 patients (14 with schizophrenia, 6 with organic brain syndrome, 3 of those 6 with alcoholism) with polydipsia (7–43 L of water per day) and hyponatremia (serum sodium concentration 98–124 mmol/L) followed for up to 28 months. Complications of hyponatremia included hypertension, headache, lethargy, seizures, coma, dementia, and death. The investigators studied seven patients after voluntary water loading. At the end of water loading when serial plasma osmolalities were 226, 242, 244, 266, 238, 238, and 244 mOsm/kg, urine osmolalities were 102, 56, 68, 87, 61, 47, and 37 mOsm/kg, respectively. At least five of these seven patients failed to maximally dilute their urine (that is, failed to achieve a urine osmolality of 50 mOsm/kg), consistent with the syndrome of inappropriate antidiuresis (Bartter and Schwartz 1967). Hariprasad et al. (1980) also showed that patients with polydipsia-hyponatremia syndrome (and the syndrome of inappropriate antidiuresis) may have urine sodium concentrations of < 20 mmol/L, contrasted with the usual patient with the syndrome of inappropriate antidiuresis who has urine sodium concentration of > 20 mmol/L (Berl et al. 1976). The large daily fluid intake leading to very dilute urine accounts for this observation. Finally, the authors noted a 10% mortality from water intoxication over 2 years in their study population.

Investigators continued to define normal urine dilution as the capacity to reduce urine osmolality to < 100 mOsm/kg. This definition led to erroneous conclusions in the literature (DeFronzo et al. 1976; Gillum and Linas 1984). Miller and Moses (1977) showed that persons can normally reduce urine osmolalities to < 40 mOsm/kg when maximally water loaded. (Based on my clinical observations, patients with polydipsia-hyponatremia syndrome can dilute their urine osmolalities to < 30 mOsm/kg under certain conditions of maximum water loading and when their circulating levels of arginine vasopressin are low but still measurable.)

Vasopressin Measurements in Patients With Polydipsia-Hyponatremia Syndrome

A study by M. B. Goldman et al. (1988) is discussed in Chapter 5. Briefly, the results of water loading and hypertonic saline infusions in a group of polydipsic-hyponatremic patients (seven with schizophrenia and one with organic delusional syndrome) and a matched patient control sample were compared. Patients with polydipsia-hyponatremia syndrome had lower basal plasma osmolality and vasopressin values than control subjects. Plasma osmolality dropped in both groups with water loading, but vasopressin showed greater reductions in the control subjects than in the polydipsic-hyponatremic patients. Estimated water desired, an approximation of thirst, tended to remain higher for patients than control subjects during water loading. Control subjects achieved a more dilute urine with water loading, and urine osmolality was consistently lower in the control group than in the polydipsic-hyponatremic patients.

Both patients and control subjects increased their plasma osmolality and vasopressin values during hypertonic saline infusion (M. B. Goldman et al. 1988). These values, however, were lower for patients than control subjects. The slope of vasopressin increase was greater for control subjects than patients. During hypertonic saline infusion, patients tended to desire more water than control subjects. The authors concluded that patients with polydipsia-hyponatremia syndrome fail to maximally dilute their urine, osmotically regulate water intake, and secrete vasopressin appropriately.

Vieweg et al. (1988j) studied the diurnal variation of water balance in seven schizophrenic patients. They measured serum sodium, plasma vasopressin, and urine osmolality weekly for 8 weeks at 7 A.M. and 4 P.M. Serum sodium concentration was normal in the morning and low in the afternoon. Vasopressin levels were lower in the afternoon than in the morning but were not appropriately suppressed despite the low afternoon serum sodium concentrations (Figure 1–1). Despite serum hypotonicity, urine was not maximally dilute (afternoon urine osmolality measurements were > 50 mOsm/kg). The authors concluded that the combination of polydipsia and abnormal vasopressin regulation contributed importantly to afternoon hyponatremia in polydipsic-hyponatremic patients (Figure 1–2).

Schizophrenic patients with polydipsia-hyponatremia syndrome consume large quantities of water and usually have low, but detectable, vasopressin levels. Patients with the syndrome of inappropriate antidiuresis described by Bartter and Schwartz (1967) consume smaller (but more than necessary) quantities of water and have greater vasopressin levels than do polydipsic-hyponatremic patients. Thus, the combination of water consumption and circulating vasopressin are the major factors leading to dilutional hyponatremia and water intoxication. The more water consumed, the lower the vasopressin concentration may be to develop water intoxication; the greater the vasopressin concentration, the lower water consumption can be to induce water intoxication (Figure 1–2). Among polydipsic-hyponatremic schizophrenic patients, we do not know whether the abnormal interplay of vasopressin and polydipsia is a state or trait phenomenon of psychosis.

Emsley et al. (1989) administered a standard water load to 23 unmedicated and nonsmoking patients with schizophrenia or schizoaffective disorder and 28 people in the control group. Neither patients nor control subjects were polydipsic. Patients had lower urine volumes and had more concentrated urine than did control subjects. That is, nonpolydipsic schizophrenic patients failed to maximally dilute their urine. This article suggested that osmotic dysregulation may be independent of chronic polydipsia in the psychoses.

Delva et al. (1990) measured plasma vasopressin, serum sodium concentration and osmolality, urine volume, vasopressin, osmolality, and creatinine in 12 polydipsic inpatients, 10 of whom had

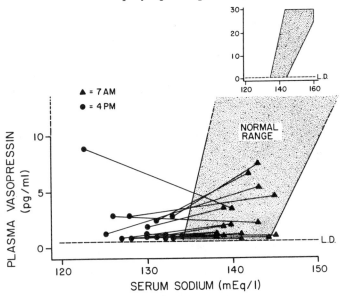

Figure 1–1.   Relationship between serum sodium and plasma vasopressin concentration at 7 A.M. and 4 P.M. in 18 samples from seven schizophrenic patients with the polydipsia-hyponatremia syndrome. Shaded areas indicate the range of normal.

Source.   Vieweg et al. 1988j. Used with permission.

Mechanism of Hyponatremia

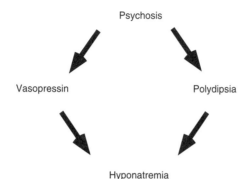

Figure 1–2. Major factors leading to dilutional hyponatremia among schizophrenic patients with polydipsia–hyponatremia syndrome.

schizophrenia. Subjects were evaluated while drinking ad libitum and then after fasting. Nine subjects showed inappropriately high plasma vasopressin levels for the degree of serum hypotonicity. Using Robertson's classification (Zerbe et al. 1980), seven subjects had type I syndrome of inappropriate antidiuresis (no relationship between plasma vasopressin and serum osmolality), and two subjects had type II syndrome of inappropriate antidiuresis (reset osmostat). The authors concluded that plasma vasopressin plus polydipsia are the main determinants of dilutional hyponatremia in patients with polydipsia-hyponatremia syndrome.

Prevalence of Polydipsia and Water Intoxication

Using nursing staff interview and chart review, Jose and Perez-Cruet (1979) reported a 6.6% prevalence of polydipsia and a 3.3% prevalence of water intoxication among 239 chronically psychotic patients (83% with schizophrenia) in a state mental hospital. Jos et al. (1986) (Jose dropped the *e* from his last name), again using nursing staff interview and chart review, identified a 6.2% prevalence of polydipsia and a 1.5% prevalence of previous water intoxication among 2,201 psychiatric patients in public hospitals or adult care facilities in St. Louis, Missouri. Among the 34 patients with a history of water intoxication, 53% were men and 85% carried a diagnosis of schizophrenia.

Using a urine specific gravity of 1.008 or less to define polydipsia, Blum and Friedland (1983) reported a 17.5% prevalence of polydipsia among 241 chronically psychotic male inpatients. Godleski et al. (1988), using an early morning urine specific gravity of 1.008 or less to define polyuria, reported a 59% prevalence of polyuria among 34 male patients (74% with chronic schizophrenia) at a state mental hospital long-term unit.

After collecting 24-hour urine volumes, Lawson et al. (1985) reported a 20% prevalence of polyuria among 35 drug-free inpatients with chronic schizophrenia. The authors did not catheterize their patients and may have underestimated urine volumes (Lawson 1986; Vieweg and David 1986). Hoskins and colleagues (Sleeper 1935) reported a 55% prevalence of urine volumes exceeding 2,000 ml per day in catheterized chronic schizophrenic inpatients.

Assessing Polyuria

Quantitating polyuria in schizophrenics dates to Hoskins and colleagues' efforts (Hoskins 1933; Hoskins and Sleeper 1933; Sleeper 1935; Sleeper and Jellinek 1936). Patients studied by Hoskins and colleagues underwent catheterization. The authors found that chronic schizophrenic inpatients excreted daily urine volumes of $2,602 \pm 1,851$ ml (range 510–8000 ml) compared with normal values of $1,328 \pm 629$ ml (range 655–2805 ml).

More than 50 years after Hoskins' work, Koczapski et al. (1989) developed a method to estimate daily fluid intake in patients with polydipsia-hyponatremia syndrome. These investigators collected 24-hour urine volumes (without catheterization) in 14 male schizophrenic patients with polydipsia (mean 9 L per day, range 3–15 L per day). They measured total urine creatinine, urine creatinine concentration at 8 A.M. (UCR1 in milligrams per deciliter) and 4 P.M. (UCR2 in milligrams per deciliter), and body weight at 8 A.M. (WT in kilograms). From this, they derived formulas to estimate daily urine volume (DUV). DUV (in liters per 24 hours for men) $= 0.875 \times ([WT \div UCR1] = [WT \div UCR2])$. For example, a male patient weighing 70 kg with UCR1 = 36 mg/dl and UCR2 = 20 mg/dl,

DUV = 0.875 x ([70 ÷ 36] + [70 ÷ 20]) = 0.875 x (1.94 + 3.5) = 4.8 L. For women, the coefficient 0.625 replaces 0.875. When SI units (mmol/L) are used to express urine creatinine concentration, the coefficients for men and women are 0.0774 and 0.0553, respectively. The coefficients for men and women differ because of gender differences in lean body mass (muscle mass).

Vieweg et al. (1984c, 1985a, 1985b, 1985d, 1985e, 1986a, 1986b, 1986c, 1988a, 1988b, 1988e, 1988f, 1988i, 1989d, 1991a) initially used morning body weight and then morning and afternoon urine creatinine concentrations to estimate daily urine volume. Recently, they compared their method (Vieweg et al. 1992a) to that of Koczapski et al. (1989).

The estimate of daily urine creatinine excretion used by Vieweg at al. (1992a) derived from the work of Kirschenbaum (1978). This investigator reported that the daily urine creatinine excretion was 15–25 mg/kg of body weight for men and 10–20 mg/kg of body weight for women. Vieweg et al. (1992a) use 20 mg/kg of morning body weight for men and 15 mg/kg of morning body weight for women to estimate daily urine creatinine excretion. The daily urine creatinine excretion of 20 mg/kg of body weight for men closely approximated Hoskins and Sleeper's (1933) findings of 19.7 mg/kg of body weight for men with chronic schizophrenia. Vieweg et al. (1992a) averaged diurnal urine creatinine concentrations (at least one morning and one afternoon measurement) to derive mean urine creatinine concentration (MUCR). Dividing the daily urine creatinine excretion by MUCR gives DUV. For example, a man weighing 70 kg in the morning would excrete 1,400 mg of creatinine in the urine daily. If the morning urine creatinine concentration was 36 mg/dl and the afternoon urine creatinine concentration was 20 mg/dl, the MUCR would be 28 mg/dl. Then, DUV = (1,400 ÷ 28) x (100) = 50 x 100 = 5,000 ml or 5 L.

Analyzing morning weight and morning and afternoon urine creatinine concentrations for 17 male and 12 female chronically psychotic patients, Vieweg et al. (1992a) found that their method correlated highly with the method of Koczapski et al. (1989) for male ($r = 0.976$, $P < .0001$) and female ($r = 0.992$, $P < .0001$) patients. The excellent correlations between these two methods suggest that both are satisfactory in estimating DUV among chronically psychotic patients. Both methods rely on the principles that urine creatinine excretion is constant and is a linear function of body weight and that excretion varies by gender. These principles are generally true, although exceptions may occur (Bleiler and Schedl 1962; Narayanan and Appleton 1980; J. P. Peters and Van Slyke 1946; Vestergaard and Leverett 1958). The more urine samples one obtains to estimate MUCR and the greater their dispersion throughout the day, the better one approximates actual daily urine volume in these calculations.

M. B. Goldman et al. (1992b) offered yet a third method to estimate DUV in chronically psychotic patients. They collected DUV (without catheterization) in 5 female and 13 male psychiatric patients. Mean 24-hour urine creatinine excretion was 22.3 mg/kg for men and 13.8 mg/kg for women. Their initial model for men and women embraced the model of Koczapski et al. (1989) for men: DUV in liters per 24 hours = 0.875 x ([WT ÷ UCR1] = [WT ÷ UCR2]). The strength of association between the two models was R^2 = 0.85. Adding gender improved the model fit. Adding age or antipsychotic drug dose did not improve the fit.

To estimate DUV for men and women, M. B. Goldman et al. (1992b) derived the equation LN(DUV in ml) = 7.2 + 0.68 (LN [weight in kg ÷ UCR at 4 P.M. in mg/dl + weight in kg ÷ UCR at 7:30 A.M.]) = 0.44 x (gender), where LN = natural logarithm and gender = 1 for men and 0 for women. This method may be harder to use in estimating DUV than the two earlier methods described. The authors asserted that spot urine samples provide an accurate estimate of DUV. Morning samples may be less predictive than afternoon samples. Morning and afternoon samples combined predict DUV.

Using the principles previously described (Vieweg et al. 1985c, 1988b, 1992b), Vieweg et al. documented the relationship between urine specific gravity and urine osmolality. They related urine specific gravity and estimated daily urine volume among psychiatric patients including those with polydipsia-hyponatremia syndrome. Urine specific gravity and urine osmolality related linearly (Vieweg et al. 1988b). For men, urine osmolality = 37267.0 x specific gravity – 37269.0. For women, urine osmolality = 33985.0 x specific gravity – 33977.4. Vieweg et al. (1988b) published an idealized tabulation of daily urine volumes by early morning urine specific gravity for a 70-kg male and a 60-kg female patient with polydipsia-hyponatremia syndrome (Table 1–1).

Corcoran (1955) noted that the strongest correlation between urine specific gravity and urine osmolality occurred when the urine sodium concentration was low secondary to a sodium-restricted diet. In that study, the correlation ranged between 0.89 on an unrestricted sodium diet and 0.96 on a 1- to 2-g sodium restricted diet.

Vieweg et al. (1988f) defined polyuria for a 70-kg man as daily urine volume exceeding 2,600 ml. For a 60-kg woman, this value was 2,200 ml. These definitions provide a useful value of 37 ml/kg of body weight for both men and women as the upper limit of normal daily urine volume. M. Goldman (1991) used 3,000 ml as the upper limit of normal daily urine volume for men and women.

NORMALIZED DIURNAL WEIGHT GAIN

In a carefully controlled metabolic study, Davidson et al. (1976) reported that healthy control-group subjects gained 0.76% ± 0.16% of their 8 A.M. weight by 4 P.M. This value compared favorably to normal values derived by Vieweg et al. (1988d). These investigators reported that normal men gained 0.60% ± 0.39% of their 7 A.M. weight by 4 P.M. For normal women, this value was 0.47% ± 0.31%. Using two standard deviations above the mean, Vieweg et al. (1988d) recommended a value of 1.2% as the upper limit of normal weight gain between 7 A.M. and 4 P.M. for men and women.

Weight Gain in Dilutional Hyponatremia

Rowntree and his group (Rowntree 1922, 1923; Weir et al. 1922) showed that weight gain occurred in dilutional hyponatremia and water intoxication. In animal experiments, they showed that the range of animal weight gain at death as a fraction of initial weight was 8.0%–26.3% for rabbits, 9.7%–52.2% for guinea pigs, and 12.0%–50.0% for cats. For a 70-kg man, the range of weight gains from *onset of water loading until death* would be 5.6–18.4 kg, 6.8–36.8 kg, and 8.4–35.0 kg, respectively. Later, Barlow and De Wardener (1959) showed weight gain in humans who continued to drink fluids after parenteral vasopressin administration.

Table 1–1. Idealized tabulation of daily urine volumes by early morning urinary specific gravities for a 70-kg male and a 60-kg female patient with polydipsia–hyponatremia syndrome

Early morning urinary specific gravity	Daily urine volume (L)	
	Male patient	Female patient
1.001	15.5 (8–23.5)	10.5 (5.5–15.5)
1.002	12.5 (5.5–20)	8 (3.5–13)
1.003	9 (4–14)	6 (2.5–9.5)
1.004	7 (2–12.5)	5 (1.5–9)
1.005	6 (2–9.5)	3.5 (1–5.5)
1.006	4.5 (2–7)	3 (1–4.5)
1.007	4 (1.5–6.5)	2.5 (1–3.5)
1.008	3 (1.5–4.5)	2 (1–3)

Adapted from Vieweg et al. 1988b. Values in parentheses are ranges.

Assessing Weight Variation in Dilutional Hyponatremia and Water Intoxication

Weight measurements of patients with polydipsia-hyponatremia syndrome is a methodology of considerable interest and importance that allows individual and group comparisons of diurnal weight variations and fluid balance monitoring of patients at risk for the development of water intoxication.

Koczapski et al. (1985) described mean diurnal (morning to afternoon) body weight gain of 4.0 kg in nine patients with recurrent water intoxication. Two years later, M. B. Goldman and Luchins (1987) recommended a target-weight procedure to monitor patients with dilutional hyponatremia. Initially, the investigators (M. Goldman 1991) established an upper weight and an upper serum sodium-concentration limit for each patient by simultaneously measuring body weight and serum sodium concentration four times over 2 weeks. They averaged each parameter to obtain mean body weight and mean serum sodium concentration. If mean serum sodium concentration was > 132 mmol/L, they set the patient's lower serum sodium concentration limit at 125 mmol/L. If mean serum sodium concentration was < 132 mmol/L, the authors set the lower limit of serum sodium concentration at mean serum sodium concentration minus 7 mmol/L. The authors calculated the patient's upper weight limit (UWL) by dividing the mean serum sodium concentration (MSS) by the lower serum sodium concentration limit (LSL) and multiplying the result by the mean body weight (MBW). That is, UWL = (MSS ÷ LSL) x MBW. For example, MSS = 133 mmol/L, LSL = 125 mmol/L, and MBW = 70 kg. Then, UWL = (133 ÷ 125) x 70 = 74.5 kg.

Vieweg et al. (1987a) offered a variation of the methods of Koczapski et al. (1985) and M. B. Goldman and Luchins (1987). Vieweg et al. (1987a) focused on percentage weight gain between 7 A.M. and 4 P.M. among chronically psychotic patients with dilutional hyponatremia subject to recurrent water intoxication.

Normalized Diurnal Weight Gain

Vieweg et al. (1988d) recommended that we use normalized diurnal weight gain (NDWG) (Figure 1–3) to assess water imbalance among chronically psychotic patients. A standard hospital counterweight scale (not a spring-loaded bathroom scale) is used. The clinician weighs the patient in the same state of dress at 7 A.M. (before breakfast) and 4 P.M. (4 hours after lunch and before dinner). The patient should void before each weighing. If residual urine volume is present after voiding, the patient (alone or helped by an attendant) uses a variation of the Credé maneuver to apply pressure above the bladder to empty it. On occasion, the clinician must catheterize the patient to ensure an empty bladder. Weighing the patient whose bladder is empty is important. Patients with recurrent water intoxication can have residual bladder volumes of 3 L or more (3 kg or 6.6 pounds or more). After accurately weighing the patient, we obtain NDWG (Figure 1–3) by subtracting 7 A.M. weight from 4 P.M. weight, dividing the difference by 7 A.M. weight, and multiplying the result by 100 to convert to a percentage. For example, 7 A.M. weight = 70 kg; 4 P.M. weight = 73.5 kg. Then, NDWG = ([73.5 – 70] ÷ 70) x 100 = 5%. That is, the patient's afternoon weight is 5% greater than the morning weight. Dividing the difference between afternoon and morning weight by the morning weight normalizes diurnal weight change so that one can compare patients with different baseline weights. The upper limit of normal for NDWG is 1.2%.

Normalized Diurnal Weight Gain in Chronic Psychosis

Delva and Crammer (1988) described eight polydipsic patients excreting up to 22 L each day. During the day, changes in plasma sodium concentration were proportional to changes in body weight. During the night patients excreted retained excess water, returning to baseline weight by morning. The authors noted that subjects who gained more than 7% of baseline weight had plasma sodium concentrations < 125 mmol/L.

Vieweg and colleagues (Vieweg et al. 1988c, 1988d, 1988e, 1988f, 1988g, 1988h, 1989a, 1989b, 1989c, 1989d, 1989e, 1989f, 1990c, 1990d, 1991a) used NDWG to survey water imbalance in chronic psychosis. Among state mental hospital patients with chronic schizophrenia, they found that 70% of patients had abnormally high NDWG. This percentage of patients with water imbalance was greater than in two earlier studies (Vieweg et al. 1986a, Godleski et al. 1988) describing the prevalence of polyuria among similar patients. In the first of the two reports, 36% of male and 45% of female patients were polyuric. In the second study, they found that 60% of chronically psychotic men (mostly with schizophrenia) were polyuric. In that NDWG reflects failure of maximal urine dilution (that is, fluid retention), it is probably a better index of water imbalance than is simple polyuria. Thus, more than two-thirds of patients with a

Normalized diurnal weight gain (NDWG)

$$\text{NDWG} = 100 \times \frac{4 \text{ P.M. weight} - 7 \text{ A.M. weight}}{7 \text{ A.M. weight}}$$

Figure 1–3.   Derivation of normalized diurnal weight gain (NDWG). Using a standard hospital counterweight scale, the clinician weighs the patient in the same state of dress at 7 A.M. (before breakfast) and 4 P.M. (4 hours after lunch and before dinner). The patient's bladder should be empty at each weighing.

chronic schizophrenic disorder requiring long-term hospitalization manifest some degree of water imbalance. Water imbalance may be an intrinsic feature of chronic schizophrenia with only the severest forms of imbalance evident clinically. In a study of 29 chronically psychotic patients (mostly with schizophrenia or schizoaffective disorder), mean NDWG was 3.1% ± 1.5% for men and 1.9% ± 0.8% for women (Vieweg et al. 1988c).

In a study of 31 chronically psychotic patients taking lithium and 42 chronically psychotic subjects not taking lithium (control subjects), Vieweg et al. (1988f) showed that NDWG was abnormal among patients and control subjects independent of lithium administration. These investigators (Vieweg et al. 1988g, 1990d) found that seasonal variation was absent in NDWG or polyuria among chronically psychotic patients. This supports Hoskins and colleagues' (Sleeper 1935) earlier observation that polyuria is stable over time in chronic schizophrenia.

Vieweg et al. (1988h, 1990c) showed that NDWG predicted change in serum sodium concentration in patients with polydipsia-hyponatremia syndrome. Vieweg et al. (1988h) used a nomogram (Figure 1–4) to predict critical afternoon serum sodium concentrations based on afternoon weight gain. Nursing staff can use this nomogram to monitor patients subject to water intoxication. Although NDWG predicts changes in serum sodium concentration, it is a less useful index of polydipsia and polyuria (Vieweg et al. 1988e, 1989d, 1991a) with correlations between NDWG and urine volume ranging between 0.36 and 0.90. The major reason for this correlation variation is that patients usually drink more fluids than they excrete in the afternoon.

Lithium and carbamazepine have opposing effects on renal action of vasopressin. Lithium alone, carbamazepine alone, or the combination of lithium and carbamazepine appear not to alter NDWG findings among patients with afternoon dilutional hyponatremia (Vieweg et al. 1989b). Also, there is usually a poor correlation between antipsychotic drugs and NDWG among chronically psychotic inpatients (Vieweg et al. 1989c).

Studying NDWG findings in chronic psychosis, Vieweg et al. (1989a) reported that about 7% of chronically psychotic long-term inpatients (most with schizophrenia) have recurrent wa-

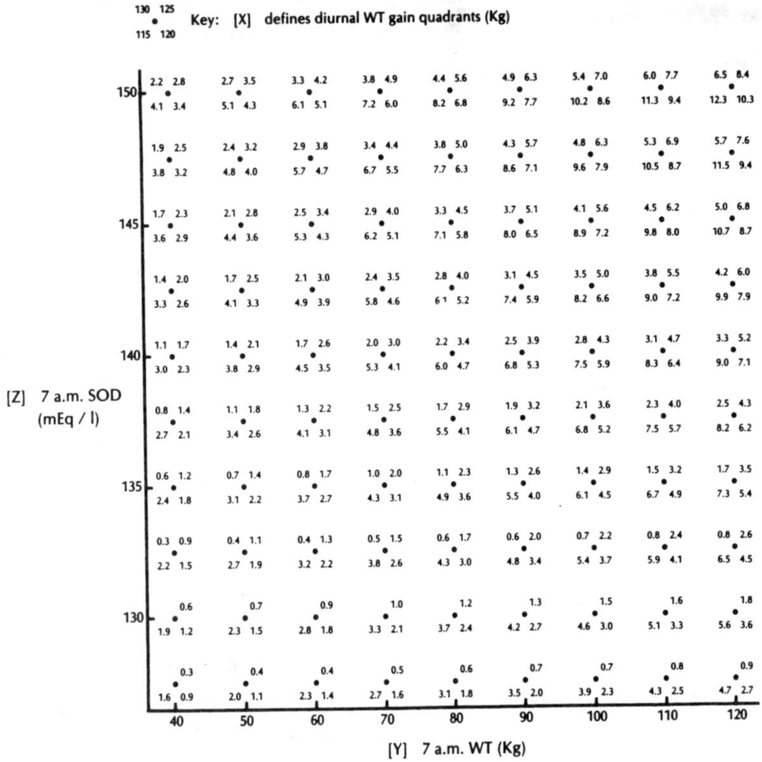

Figure 1–4. Tabulation of the relationship between antidiuresis and hyponatremia in the polydipsia-hyponatremia syndrome. The key (left upper corner) defines four quadrants of 4 P.M. serum sodium concentrations associated with the diurnal weight gain (baseline 7 A.M. weight) in kg necessary to produce 4 P.M. serum sodium concentrations of 130, 125, 120, and 115 mmol/ L. For example, a patient whose 7 A.M. measurements of weight (WT) and serum sodium concentration (SOD) were 80 kg (176 pounds) and 140 mmol/ L, respectively, would have 4 P.M. SOD levels of 130, 125, 120, and 115 mmol/ L with 4 P.M. WT gains of 2.2 kg (4.8 pounds), 3.4 kg (7.5 pounds), 4.7 kg (10.3 pounds), and 6.0 kg (13.2 pounds), respectively.
Source.   Reprinted from Vieweg et al. 1988h. Used with permission.

ter intoxication and an additional 60% have abnormally high NDWG without evidence of recurrent water intoxication. Extending these findings, water dysregulation appears to develop during the chronic stage of schizophrenia (Vieweg et al. 1989f) independent of antipsychotic drug dose. Acutely psychotic patients have NDWG values not statistically different from the general population.

Course in Polydipsia-Hyponatremia Syndrome

Patients with schizophrenia destined to develop polydipsia-hyponatremia syndrome are indistinguishable from other patients with schizophrenia at the onset of their illness (Vieweg et al. 1984a, 1984d). They develop psychosis in late adolescence or their early 20s. At this stage, parameters of water regulation are normal. A clinically silent period of 5–15 years starts during which time health care professionals consider patients to be metabolically stable. In retrospect, polydipsia and polyuria emerge as seen by progressively more dilute spot urine specific gravities. Singh et al. (1985) stated that psychiatric patients with a urine specific gravity of < 1.008 and a history of polyuria should have their water intake monitored and serum electrolytes evaluated. Besides using a low urine specific gravity to identify patients at risk for water intoxication, the authors noted that low blood-urea nitrogen (< 6 mg/dl) was common when dilutional hyponatremia accompanied hyposthenuria. Characteristically, patients developing polydipsia-hyponatremia syndrome are first noted to be polydipsic in their early 30s. In their mid-30s, they present with severe hyposthenuria (urine specific gravity of ≤ 1.003) and generalized seizures secondary to water intoxication.

A generalized seizure is the first recognized problem in patients with polydipsia-hyponatremia syndrome in more than 80% of cases (Jos 1984; Jose et al. 1979; Jose and Evenson 1980; Vieweg et al. 1984a). The review by Jose and Evenson (1980) of cases of psychosis and water intoxication found 44 cases with the first one noted in 1938 (Barahal 1938). The mean age was 42 years, and 61% were women. In a subset of 13 patients studied by the authors, the mean age was 41 years, and all were non-Hispanic whites. The mean time between onset of psychosis and first episode of water intoxication was 19 years, and the mean serum sodium concentration when water intoxicated was 119 mmol/L.

Complications in Polydipsia-Hyponatremia Syndrome

Until the late 1930s, clinicians and investigators considered polydipsia a benign process in humans, although Rowntree and colleagues (Rowntree 1922, 1923; Weir et al. 1922) had ably documented the many complications of water intoxication in animals. Complications of recurrent water intoxication divide into those more closely related to polydipsia and those more closely related to hyponatremia (Table 1–2).

Arieff et al. (1976) found that plasma sodium concentration correlated well with level of consciousness and presence of generalized seizures in 66 hyponatremic patients. Of 14 patients with acute hyponatremia (less than 12 hours duration) the mean plasma sodium was 112 mmol/L. All had decreased levels of consciousness and four had generalized seizures. Five of these patients died. In cases where hyponatremia lasted at least 3 days, mean plasma

Table 1–2. Complications occurring in psychotic patients associated with recurrent water intoxication divided into those most closely related to polydipsia and those most closely related to hyponatremia

Polydipsia	Hyponatremia
Polyuria	Delirium
Hypocalcemia	Worsening psychosis
Hypercalciuria	Generalized seizures
Osteopenia	Coma
Bone fractures	Death
Dilated and hypotonic bowel and bladder	
Malabsorption	
Hydronephrosis	
Renal failure	
Congestive heart failure	

sodium concentration was 115 mmol/L among those with symptoms and 122 mmol/L among those without symptoms. Among those with symptoms, 8% had seizures and 12% died. None of the asymptomatic patients had seizures or died.

In addition, Arieff et al. (1976) reported that if plasma sodium concentration was < 125 mmol/L in asymptomatic animals, subclinical brain edema ensued. Subclinical brain edema may progress to permanent brain damage. The authors recommended that patients, particularly if symptomatic, with plasma sodium concentrations of < 125 mmol/L receive hypertonic saline infusions.

Vieweg et al. (1985a) showed that water intoxication was a common cause of death in 60 middle-aged state mental hospital patients. Of these, 27 (45%) suffered from schizophrenia and five (18.5%) died from water intoxication. The authors compared their findings to earlier reports of death as a result of water intoxication among patients with schizophrenia (Blotcky et al. 1980; DiMaio and DiMaio 1980; Raskind 1974; Rendell et al. 1978). Common clinical features included psychosis, polydipsia, polyuria, severe hyposthenuria (urine specific gravity of < 1.003), hyponatremia (94–120 mmol/L), seizures, coma, and cerebral and visceral edema. When premortem findings of polydipsia and hyponatremia are not available, evidence of antecedent severe hyposthenuria and postmortem vitreous-humor hyponatremia of < 120 mmol/L strongly support the diagnosis of death caused by water intoxication.

Thiazide diuretics, tolbutamide, and carbamazepine have been shown to enhance the risk of water intoxication in psychotic patients with polydipsia-hyponatremia syndrome (R. A. Emsley et al. 1990; Levine et al. 1987; Peh et al. 1990). Such drugs should be used cautiously in polydipsic patients.

Other long-term complications of polydipsia-hyponatremia include hypotonic bladder and hydronephrosis (Blum and Friedland 1983; Harrison et al. 1979; Moskowitz 1992). Chronic overdistension (megacystis) is the mechanism limiting urine excretion. Residual urine volumes may reach 3 L. Renal failure and death may follow. Treatment includes initial indwelling catheter drainage (sometimes for up to 2 months) to decompress the bladder and regain muscle tone.

Mild to moderate hypocalcemia also occurs in patients with polydipsia-hyponatremia syndrome (Vieweg et al. 1986d). Delva et al. (1989) extended these observations of calcium dysregulation in patients with polydipsia-hyponatremia syndrome to include osteopenia, pathological fractures, and hypercalciuria. Serum calcium, alkaline phosphatase, liver function testing, renal function testing, and hematological parameters were normal. Cortisol, testosterone, estradiol, and luteinizing hormone levels were normal. Phosphate, thyroxine, and follicle-stimulating hormone were increased in polydipsic patients. They concluded that extracellular space expansion contributed to hypercalciuria and attendant skeletal changes.

Water Imbalance Is Not Specific to Schizophrenia

Besides patients with schizophrenia and schizoaffective disorder, patients with mental retardation (Vieweg et al. 1989h), dementia (Vieweg et al. 1989g), and bipolar spectrum disorder (Vieweg et al. 1990b) may have abnormally high NDWG measurements. Mentally retarded patients had fewer abnormally high NDWG values compared with subjects suffering from organic mental syndromes (Vieweg et al. 1989h). Central nervous system injury occurs earlier in mental retardation than among subjects with organic mental disorders. The timing of central nervous system injury may influence the frequency and the severity of water imbalance. These findings provide additional evidence separating patients with mental retardation from those with organic psychosis.

Additional studies have shown that water imbalance occurs in disorders other than schizophrenia and schizoaffective disorder. Jose and Perez-Cruet (1979), Bremner and Regan (1991), and Shah and Greenberg (1992) reported water imbalance in mental retardation. Patients with dementia and water imbalance have been reported by Jos et al. (1986) and Tallis (1989). Brown et al. (1983), Zubenko et al. (1984), Crammer (1986), and Jos et al. (1986) reported water imbalance in affective disorders, including bipolar disorder. Among compulsive water drinkers reported by Barlow and De Wardener (1959), psychiatric diagnoses included depression, hysteria, bulimia, and delusional hypochondriasis. Santy and Schwartz (1983) described a patient with a lung abscess, dilutional hyponatremia, and acute mania.

MANAGING POLYDIPSIA-HYPONATREMIA SYNDROME

Until the 1930s, clinicians considered polydipsia and polyuria to be benign phenomena among psychiatric patients (Hoskins 1933). Physicians tried to distinguish between polydipsia and polyuria associated with psychiatric conditions from the polydipsia and polyuria of diabetes insipidus (Bauer 1925). After clinicians diagnosed diabetes insipidus, they prescribed vasopressin as replacement therapy. In the first reported case of schizophrenia and water intoxication (Barahal 1938), seizure treatment was limited to observation and bromide and chloral hydrate administration via stomach tube. Barlow and De Wardener (1959) used treatments including continuous narcosis, electroconvulsive therapy, and reassurance among their patients with compulsive water drinking. Hobson and English (1963), in their study of a schizophrenic patient with the syndrome of inappropriate antidiuresis, asserted that fluid restriction alone can restore normal serum sodium concentration. The authors discouraged treating such patients with supplemental salt.

Fluid Restriction

Bartter and Schwartz (1967) restricted fluid intake to 500–700 ml per day to achieve a total weight loss of 2–4 kg among patients with syndrome of inappropriate antidiuresis. Fluid restriction remains the cornerstone of treating psychiatric patients with polydipsia-hyponatremia syndrome (Godleski et al. 1989; M. Goldman 1991; Illowsky and Kirch 1988; Lapierre et al. 1990; A. T. Riggs et al. 1991; and Zubenko 1987). This intervention, either voluntary or imposed, is not always successful, particularly among chronically psychotic patients. In part, this is because some schizophrenic patients with polydipsia-hyponatremia syndrome say they drink water to feel better (Millson et al. 1989).

Change in Serum Sodium Concentration as a Determinant of Water Intoxication

Koczapski and Millson (1989) studied eight schizophrenic men with polydipsia-hyponatremia syndrome for 1 year. Serial measurements showed that the magnitude and rate of change in serum sodium concentration, not its absolute level, best explain the severity of symptoms and signs in water intoxication. Thus, to prevent water intoxication, clinicians should follow changes in water balance parameters to protect against water intoxication rather than dictating intervention based on absolute serum sodium concentration.

Vasopressin and Chronic Psychosis

Investigators have used vasopressin (known to influence learning, memory, and behavior) to treat psychotic patients. J. R. E. Davis et al. (1981) described a 63-year-old woman with bipolar disorder admitted because of an acute hypomanic episode. Without lithium therapy, she excreted 5-6 L of urine per day. To test for diabetes insipidus, she received 4 µg of DDAVP intramuscularly in the evening. Polydipsia continued. That night she became comatose with decorticate posture. Serum sodium concentration was 114 mmol/L. She received intravenous hypertonic saline and recovered 14 hours later. The authors pointed out the hazards of giving vasopressin to polydipsic patients.

Raskind et al. (1978) indicated that plasma vasopressin, measured by radioimmunoassay, was higher in acutely psychotic patients than in acutely anxious nonpsychotic patients or control subjects. Vasopressin levels correlated positively with the degree of psychosis. Despite elevated vasopressin measurements in acutely psychotic patients, serum sodium determinations were normal. This is not surprising because none of the acutely psychotic patients was polydipsic. Vasopressin levels were normal in the anxious nonpsychotic patients.

Group Psychotherapy

Using principles employed to treat schizophrenic outpatients with substance abuse (Hellerstein and Meehan 1987; Kofoed et al. 1986),

Millson et al. (1993) conducted a controlled, prospective 4-month group psychotherapy study of 10 male schizophrenic inpatients with polydipsia-hyponatremia syndrome. The authors matched subjects by diurnal changes in body weight, Mini-Mental State Exam score, and Brief Psychiatric Rating Scale score. They then randomly assigned study subjects either to group psychotherapy or control status for the 4-month study. Group psychotherapy was two weekly 45-minute sessions of mainly psychoeducational material. Group leaders used art therapy to help patients focus on excessive fluid intake and to initiate self-disclosure. They showed patients the relationship between water consumption and weight gain by first asking them to fill a 4 L jug with water. Patients then measured their weight holding and not holding the 4 L jug. The authors also helped the patients to count the number of cups of water in the 4 L container. They encouraged the patients to drink no more cups each day than the 4 L container held. In addition, the risks of polydipsia, including seizures, were described with the aid of medical charts, and the mechanics of bladder distention were demonstrated using water-filled balloons.

The five polydipsic-hyponatremic patients receiving group psychotherapy drank significantly less fluid and had reduced diurnal weight gain than did the control subjects. However, once the authors stopped group psychotherapy, study subjects rapidly resumed their polydipsic behavior. Millson et al. (1993) pointed out the success of group psychotherapy in polydipsic-hyponatremic patients and the need to continue such treatment indefinitely.

A Comprehensive Treatment Approach

Clinical history remains the most important source of information to understand and treat patients with psychiatric and nonpsychiatric illnesses. Meticulous record keeping by physicians and staff caring for chronically psychotic patients is imperative because the patients are often poor historians. Family members also may provide medical and psychiatric information. Progressive water imbalance is often silent in schizophrenia until the patient suffers a generalized seizure in front of the family, spouse, neighbor, case manager, or clinical staff. Clues of emerging polydipsia and polyuria include reports of preoccupation with drinking, observed increased water consumption, nocturnal bed wetting, urinary incontinence, and worsening of the psychosis in the afternoon and early evening.

Because most patients with polydipsia-hyponatremia syndrome reside in state mental hospitals, reviewing chart laboratory data is often revealing. Whatever else may or may not be in the patient's chart or outpatient record, there usually are annual urine specific gravity measurements. Progressive hyposthenuria documents the accelerating course of polydipsia. At the onset of the patient's psychosis, morning urine specific gravity is usually greater than 1.020. This value diminishes almost annually. Once morning urine specific gravity reaches 1.008, the patient is drinking more than normal amounts of fluid. Then, the clinician should advise family, spouse, case manager, and clinical staff that the patient is at risk for water intoxication. Weigh the patient on standard hospital (counterweight) scales in the morning and the afternoon. If the patient resides at home, the family, spouse, or case manager must help the patient buy (for about $80) appropriate scales. If the patient resides in the hospital (as is usually the case), daily diurnal weight measurement should be part of the patient's treatment plan. Weigh the patient wearing the same clothes in the morning and the afternoon and have the patient void just before each weighing. The clinician following the patient should maintain a log or flow chart of daily weights.

When normalized diurnal weight gain (NDWG, Figure 1–3) exceeds 3%, consider starting the patient on the combination of lithium and phenytoin, monitoring blood levels in the usual manner (Vieweg et al. 1988k). Try to maintain lithium levels between 0.6 and 1.0 mmol/L and phenytoin levels between 10 and 20 μg/ml. Another drug treatment would be demeclocycline 300 mg tid or qid. Alternatively or concurrently, one can start a behavioral modification program to reduce polydipsia (Vieweg 1993). If the patient resides outside the hospital and the clinician cannot maintain NDWG below 3%, admit the patient to the hospital.

In the hospital, develop a target weight procedure (M. Goldman 1991; M. B. Goldman and Luchins 1987) or a NDWG procedure (Koczapski et al. 1985; Vieweg et al. 1988d). Treatment should raise morning serum sodium concentrations routinely ≥ 130 mmol/L. This effect will allow a drop in afternoon serum sodium concentration of about 10 mmol/L (occurring with NDWG of about 7% [Godleski et al. 1989]), keeping afternoon serum sodium concentration above 120 mmol/L.

As discussed in more detail by Godleski et al. (1989), Vieweg (1994), and Vieweg et al. (1994), and outlined in Table 1–3, if weight or weight change suggests a serum sodium concentration of 128–130 mmol/L, restrict the patient to the ward until the next day and limit fluid intake to less than 3 L. If weight or weight change suggests a serum sodium concentration below 128 mmol/L, measure serum sodium concentration.

If measured serum sodium concentration is 125–130 mmol/L, give 4.5 g sodium chloride (two 2.25-g tablets) by mouth, restrict the patient to the ward for medical observation, and limit fluid consumption to less than 3 L. If the measured serum sodium concentration is 120–125 mmol/L and the patient is free of symptoms and signs of water intoxication, give 4.5 g salt by mouth and repeat the dose in 2 hours. Restrict such patients to their rooms (free of water) and weigh them every 2 hours. Measure serum sodium concentration again in the morning. If the measured serum sodium concentration is 115–120 mmol/L and the patient is free of symptoms and signs of water intoxication, give 4.5 g salt by mouth and repeat the dose at 2 and 4 hours. Weigh such patients hourly until the weight corresponds to a serum sodium concentration of 125 mmol/L, restrict them to their rooms, and place them on one-to-one medical observation to ensure fluid restriction.

When the measured serum sodium concentration is below 115 mmol/L or the patient has severe symptoms or signs of water intoxication (profound agitation, change in level of consciousness, or stupor) transfer the patient to a medical center. If the patient has generalized seizures or becomes comatose, administer 3%–5% hypertonic saline intravenously, with or without supplemental intravenous furosemide (initial single dose: 1 mg/kg of body weight [Hantman et al. 1973]) over 2–3 hours trying not to raise serum sodium concentration at a rate greater than 1–2 mmol/L/hour. Almost certainly the patient's generalized seizures will stop at this point. Then, cease intravenous saline administration (even if patient remains stuporous) and limit treatment to fluid restriction and life support. There is no need to give saline to bring serum

Table 1–3. Outline of staff interventions based on estimated and measured serum sodium concentrations for patients with the polydipsia-hyponatremia syndrome

Serum sodium concentration (mmol/l)	Staff intervention
128–130 **Estimated** by weight change	Restrict patient to ward until next day and limit fluid intake to <3L per day.
<128 **Estimated** by weight change	Measure serum sodium concentration.
125–130 **Measured**	Give 4.5 g salt [two 2.25-g tablets] by mouth, restrict patient to ward for medical observation, and limit fluid consumption to <3L per day.
120–125 **Measured** Patient asymptomatic	Give 4.5 g salt by mouth and repeat dose in 2 hours. Restrict to water-free room and weigh every 2 hours. Measure serum sodium concentration again in morning.
115–120 **Measured** Patient asymptomatic	Give 4.5 g salt by mouth and repeat dose in 2 and 4 hours. Weigh patient hourly until weight corresponds to serum sodium concentration of 125 mmol/L, restrict to room, and place on one-to-one medical observation to ensure fluid restriction.
<115 **Measured** or patient has severe symptoms and signs of water intoxication	Transfer patient to a medical center. If patient has generalized seizures or becomes comatose, administer 3%–5% hypertonic saline intravenously, with or without supplemental intravenous furosemide (initial dose 1 mg/kg of body weight [Hantman et al. 1973]) over 2–3 hours trying not to raise serum sodium concentration >1–2 mmol/L/hour. Almost certainly, patient's generalized seizures will be controlled at this point. Then, stop intravenous saline administration and limit treatment to fluid restriction and life support.

sodium concentration above 120 mmol/L (Black 1989; Vieweg and Karp 1994).

Antipsychotic drugs are indicated in the treatment of polydipsia-hyponatremia syndrome. The clinician must control both water imbalance and psychosis. If the patient does not develop hypotension secondary to antipsychotic drug treatment, drug treatment will not stimulate vasopressin's release or action or worsen water-seeking behavior (Raskind et al. 1987). One antipsychotic drug is not superior to another. Side-effect profile should dictate drug selection. The claim that anticholinergic properties of antipsychotic drugs produce polydipsia seems exaggerated. The tertiary tricyclic antidepressant drugs have greater anticholinergic properties than antipsychotic drugs and, yet, we rarely find polydipsia or water imbalance in depression.

A Look Forward

Investigators have intensely studied polyuric patients over the past 100 years. At first, they tried to distinguish between idiopathic polydipsia and diabetes insipidus. Now, they incorporate the syndrome of inappropriate antidiuresis into the pathophysiology of polydipsia and dilutional hyponatremia found commonly among chronic schizophrenic patients. These insights further support the idea of schizophrenia as a neurodevelopmental or neurodegenerative process.

Techniques to study water imbalance in schizophrenia differ from the more common probes into the neocortex (electroencephalography, computerized axial tomography, and magnetic resonance imaging). By exploring more primitive central nervous structures (posterior lobe of the pituitary gland and the hypothalamus), water balance studies allow us to enter the central nervous system through the "back door." Arginine vasopressin is manufactured in the hypothalamus and travels directly to the pituitary gland posterior lobe for release. Hypothalamic-releasing factors govern pituitary gland anterior lobe hormone secretion. Studying vasopressin may be a more direct approach to the hypothalamus than investigating pituitary gland anterior lobe hormones. Vasopressin is the central nervous system hormone most consistently disturbed in schizophrenia.

Treatment of water imbalance in schizophrenia is in its infancy (Vieweg 1993; 1994; Vieweg and Karp 1994). Objective parameters to follow as we try to normalize water balance in schizophrenia include fluid intake, plasma vasopressin, serum sodium concentration and osmolality, fluid excretion, and diurnal changes in body weight. Diurnal body weight change is the most important *single* parameter to follow because it incorporates most of the other variables. Few investigators are studying this problem. Working together should be highly productive and eliminate duplicate effort. Although we can modestly alter central nervous system release or renal effect of vasopressin, polydipsia and its attendant problems persist in patients with polydipsia-hyponatremia syndrome. We need controlled trials of various drugs and their combinations that alter the release or effect of vasopressin. Perhaps, investigators may find agents binding vasopressin (antigen-antibody reaction) that we can use in humans. We must study drugs that decrease thirst.

As reviewed by Vieweg (1993), behavioral approaches to thirst disturbance offer promise but are labor intensive. If we can develop more effective and simpler behavioral treatments, the next step will probably be to prevent polydipsia-hyponatremia syndrome. Using currently available survey techniques, we can identify the onset of polydipsia and, using behavioral approaches, prevent isolated polydipsia from moving on to the more malignant polydipsia-hyponatremia syndrome.

Chapter 2

Special Topics in Water Balance in Schizophrenia

W. Victor R. Vieweg, M.D., F.A.C.P., F.A.C.C.

BODY COMPOSITION: BASELINE AND HIGH FLUID INTAKE

Application of tracer techniques has advanced our understanding of body water and electrolytes (I. S. Edelman et al. 1952; Moore 1946). Total body water as a percentage of body weight varies according to age and gender (I. S. Edelman and Leibman 1959) (Table 2–1). Body fat is greater among women, increasing with age in both men and women. Muscle mass decreases with age in both sexes. Body water distribution and body sodium distribution for a healthy young man appear in Tables 2–2 and 2–3, respectively. Thus, *plasma values* as a percentage of total body values are 7.5% for water and 11.2% for sodium in young men.

Habener et al. (1964) assessed serum and urine osmolality among control subjects who increased fluid intake progressively over 4 weeks, reaching 8.5 L per day during the fourth week. Serum osmolality did not differ from baseline when measured repeatedly in the early morning and during weekly 6.5-hour water deprivation testing. Urine osmolality progressively decreased with fluid deprivation as subjects moved through the 4-week protocol, possibly as a result of partial renal refractoriness to vasopressin or a renal medullary "washout" effect. In the last 2 weeks of the protocol, afternoon serum osmolality decreased slightly (from 7 to 21 mOsm/kg) during maximal fluid ingestion.

Table 2–1. Total body water as a percentage of body weight by age and gender

Age (yrs)	Men (%)	Women (%)
10–16	59	57
17–39	61	51
40–59	55	47
60+	52	46

Source. Adapted from I. S. Edelman and Leibman 1959.

Table 2–2. Body water distribution for a healthy young man

Compartment	Percentage
Intracellular water	55.0
Interstitial and lymph water	20.0
Plasma water	7.5
Dense connective tissue and cartilage water	7.5
Bone water	7.5
Transcellular water	2.5

Source. Adapted from I. S. Edelman and Leibman 1959.

Table 2–3. Body sodium distribution for a healthy young man

Compartment	Percentage
Total bone sodium including exchangeable bone sodium	43.1
Interstitial and lymph sodium	29.0
Plasma sodium	11.2
Dense connective tissue and cartilage sodium	11.7
Intracellular sodium	2.4
Transcellular sodium	2.6

Source. Adapted from I. S. Edelman and Leibman 1959.

These findings may have implications for patients with polydipsia-hyponatremia syndrome because they suggest that impaired output of water may result from excessive water intake. Thus, in polydipsia-hyponatremia syndrome, factors impairing renal concentrating capacity may be a consequence of long-term polydipsia and further may explain how daytime drinking could worsen hyponatremia in the afternoon.

HYPONATREMIA AND VOLUME STATE

The Colorado Group (Berl et al. 1976) classifies hyponatremia by volume state (Table 2–4). Hypovolemic hyponatremia is a deficit of total body water and larger deficit of total body sodium. Extracellular volume depletion is present. Extrarenal causes of hypovolemic hyponatremia include vomiting, diarrhea, and "third

Table 2–4.   Laboratory values and common clinical entities by volume state in hyponatremia

Laboratory values	Hypovolemia	Euvolemia	Hypervolemia
Serum sodium concentration	Decreased	Decreased	Decreased
Serum osmolality	Decreased	Decreased	Decreased
Urinary osmolality	Increased	Increased	Increased
Urinary sodium concentration	Decreased	Increased	Decreased
	< 10 mmol/L	> 20 mmol/L	< 10 mmol/L
Common clinical entities	Fever Vomiting Diarrhea	Syndrome of inappropriate antidiuresis Adrenal insufficiency Hypothyroidism Pain Emotion Drugs Psychosis	Congestive heart failure Cirrhosis with ascites Nephrotic syndrome

Source.   Berl et al. 1976.

space" problems with burns, pancreatitis, and traumatized muscle. Treatment includes isotonic saline administration.

Euvolemic hyponatremia (dilutional hyponatremia) is excess total body water and normal total body sodium. Whereas there is modest extracellular volume expansion, because there is no clinical evidence of edema, it is called *euvolemic* hyponatremia. Treatment includes fluid restriction.

Hypervolemic hyponatremia is excess total body sodium and larger excess of total body water. Extracellular volume excess with edema is clinically evident. Extrarenal causes of hypervolemic hyponatremia include congestive heart failure, cirrhosis with ascites, and the nephrotic syndrome. Treatment includes fluid restriction.

In extrarenal hyponatremic states, urine sodium concentration distinguishes euvolemic hyponatremia from hypovolemic and hypervolemic hyponatremia (Table 2–4). The urine sodium concentration is > 20 mmol/L in euvolemic hyponatremic states, consistent with syndrome of inappropriate antidiuresis. In extrarenal causes of hypovolemic and hypervolemic hyponatremia, the urine sodium concentration is characteristically < 10 mmol/L.

Serum sodium concentration may not always correlate well with serum osmolality. The presence of hyperglycemia, hyperlipidemia, and hyperproteinemia may depress sodium concentration in the serum causing "pseudohyponatremia." If serum sodium concentration is measured in these settings without concomitantly measuring serum or plasma osmolality, the clinician may misinterpret the findings. Weisberg (1989) pointed out that clinicians must be familiar with the methods used by their clinical laboratories to measure serum sodium concentrations to properly interpret these measurements.

The clinician can often distinguish among the hyponatremic volume states at the bedside. If extracellular volume depletion (hypovolemic hyponatremia) is present, blood pressure often decreases (orthostatic hypotension) and pulse increases as the patient moves between the supine and sitting or standing positions (positive tilt test). If extracellular volume excess is present (hypervolemic hyponatremia), edema is evident clinically. Without clinical evidence of hypo- or hypervolemia, the clinician assumes that euvolemic hyponatremia is present and seeks confirmation by measuring urine sodium concentration.

Recent studies point out difficulties in assessing fluid volume states in hyponatremia (Chung et al. 1987). Prospectively, the authors selected 58 nonedematous patients with serum sodium concentration of < 130 mmol/L. Clinical assessment correctly identified only about half the hypovolemic and euvolemic patients. The authors found that urine sodium concentration in spot urine samples correctly separated hypovolemic from euvolemic hyponatremic patients.

When renal disease is present, measuring urine sodium concentration does not distinguish as well among the hyponatremic volume states (Berl et al. 1976). When renal salt wasting caused by diuretic excess, mineralocorticoid deficiency, salt-losing nephritis, or renal tubular acidosis is present, urine sodium concentration is commonly > 20 mmol/L. In acute and chronic renal failure, urine sodium concentration is commonly > 20 mmol/L.

URINE EXCRETION PATTERNS IN PSYCHIATRIC PATIENTS

Hoskins and colleagues (Sleeper 1935) established that urine excretion patterns among patients with chronic schizophrenia are stable over time. Later, Vieweg et al. (1986c) looked at diurnal variation of urine excretion in patients with polydipsia-hyponatremia syndrome. Dividing the day into quarters starting at midnight, they found that patients with polydipsia-hyponatremia syndrome excrete 21.6% of their urine volume between midnight and 6 A.M.; 20.5% between 6 A.M. and 12 noon, 27.4% between 12 noon and 6 P.M.; and 30.4% of their urine volume between 6 P.M. and midnight. Thus, about 40% of the urine volume is excreted from midnight to noon and 60% between noon and midnight.

In an extension of this work (Vieweg et al. 1988i) noted that urine excretory patterns were similar for nonpolyuric and polyuric patients with chronic psychosis. That is, the slope of the change in urine creatinine concentration throughout the day and night was similar for nonpolydipsic and polydipsic men and women.

Polydipsic patients, however, excreted more urine during each quarter of the day compared with nonpolyuric patients. The authors concluded that institutionalized chronically psychotic patients respond to thirst stimuli similarly qualitatively but not quantitatively. Polydipsic patients drink more fluids at comparable times during the day than do their nonpolydipsic counterparts. A shift in thirst threshold, not such factors as hallucinations and delusions, explains polydipsic patterns in polydipsia-hyponatremia syndrome (M. B. Goldman et al. 1988; Kirch et al. 1985).

SMOKING AND ALCOHOLISM

The Colorado group (Cadnapaphornchai et al. 1974) found that nicotine increased vasopressin release by altering cervical parasympathetic tone. Rowe et al. (1980) offered another hypothesis. Using the new and highly sensitive vasopressin assay of Robertson et al. (1973), they found that intravenous nicotine administration did not affect plasma vasopressin levels. Rather, the respiratory mechanics of smoking seemed to best explain nicotine's antidiuretic action. Cigarettes with high nicotine content had higher vasopressin levels than cigarettes with low nicotine content.

Retrospectively, Gleadhill et al. (1982) studied 20,782 admissions to a university hospital's medical service. They found 172 (0.8%) cases of schizophrenia and 84 (0.36%) cases of severe dilutional hyponatremia (10 [5.8%] with schizophrenia) not caused by heart, liver, kidney, or endocrine disease. Six of the 10 schizophrenics with dilutional hyponatremia smoked more than one pack of cigarettes per day (smoking history was unknown in two patients). Statistically ($P = 0.16$), the prevalence of heavy smoking was no greater among schizophrenic patients with (75%) than those without (60%) dilutional hyponatremia. Besides his study, Blum (1984) uncovered only two reports of schizophrenic patients with dilutional hyponatremia whose hyponatremia was related to smoking. In his earlier report, Blum et al. (1983) found that all 10 patients with polydipsia-hyponatremia syndrome were heavy smokers. Vieweg et al. (1986b) found no relationship between serum nicotine levels and serum sodium concentrations among 10 patients with polydipsia-hyponatremia syndrome. The authors asserted that psychosis is a sufficiently powerful stimulus to explain thirst and osmotic disturbance in polydipsia-hyponatremia syndrome without invoking nicotine's effect on vasopressin.

Allon et al. (1990) showed that cigarette smoking impaired free-water clearance under short-term experimental conditions in six healthy subjects and two schizophrenic patients with acute dilutional hyponatremia. They induced steady-state diuresis and normal free-water clearance in control subjects and patients. Then, both groups smoked cigarettes; this action was followed promptly by impaired free-water clearance. Vieweg et al. (1991b) asserted that nicotine did not explain hyponatremia in the subjects of Allon et al. (1990) because patients and control subjects responded similarly to nicotine, 29% of the United States population smokes cigarettes, water intoxication appears almost exclusively among psychiatric patients with advanced and chronic psychosis, and there is no correlation between serum nicotine and serum sodium concentrations in patients with polydipsia-hyponatremia syndrome (Vieweg et al. 1986b).

With regard to alcoholism, Ripley et al. (1989) found alcohol abuse prevalence higher among schizophrenics with recurrent water intoxication than among matched subjects with normal water balance. Others (Blum et al. 1983; Jose and Evenson 1980; Singh et al. 1985) suggested that antecedent alcohol abuse in schizophrenia increases the risk of subsequently developing water intoxication. Recent alcohol abuse increases the risk for central pontine myelinolysis.

THE IMPACT OF AGE ON WATER BALANCE IN PSYCHOSIS

Healthy elderly men have reduced thirst after water deprivation (P.A. Phillips et al. 1984b). Because total body water decreases with age, we may not need to drink as much as we get older. P. A. Phillips et al. (1984b) concluded that diminished urine concentrating capacity occurring with age does not derive from lower vasopressin levels but reflects renal changes. Although hypodipsia may be more common among elderly people than among young people, the syndrome of inappropriate antidiuresis may relate to advanced age (C. S. Goldstein et al. 1983).

Vieweg et al. (1989g) assessed normalized diurnal weight gain among geriatric and nongeriatric psychiatric patients. They noted a lower abnormal normalized diurnal weight gain prevalence among geriatric patients with major psychiatric disorders requiring inpatient care than among their younger counterparts. Diagnoses and drugs did not explain these differences. The authors concluded that water imbalance is a risk factor for premature death among patients with chronic psychiatric illnesses. Vieweg et al. (1993) asserted that hypernatremia was a more common and serious problem than hyponatremia among elderly people requiring long-term inpatient care.

ATRIAL NATRIURETIC PEPTIDE

Changes in glomerular sodium filtration and aldosterone alone do not preserve sodium excretion at the desired level. Because sodium loading produced natriuresis after removing the first two factors (De Wardener et al. 1961), investigators postulated a third factor. Atrial natriuretic peptide, isolated from right and left atrial appendices in 1981 (de Bold 1985), is a diuretic (natriuretic), lowers blood pressure, and inhibits renin and aldosterone secretion. It contributes to short- and long-term control of water and electrolyte balance and blood pressure.

Cogan et al. (1988a; 1988b) estimated that more than 94% of serum sodium concentration decrease in dilutional hyponatremia is because of water retention. Atrial-natriuretic-peptide-induced natriuresis explained less than 6% of the decrease. The investigators explained the defect in maximal urine dilution in polydipsia-hyponatremia syndrome by vasopressin-induced antidiuresis and a decrease in solute delivery to the nephron diluting section. The second explanation derived from protracted natriuresis caused by polydipsia-induced atrial natriuretic peptide secretion, a vasopressin-independent factor (see also Vieweg and Godleski 1988b).

Vieweg et al. (1990a) showed that patients with polydipsia-hyponatremia syndrome have higher afternoon than morning atrial natriuretic peptide levels. They ascribed this difference to afternoon volume expansion. Although afternoon atrial natriuretic peptide levels are increased, afternoon vasopressin levels are decreased compared with morning measurements in this syndrome. Plasma atrial natriuretic peptide concentration may be a very sensitive volume expansion index. If so, the clinician may identify water imbalance early in the course of schizophrenia.

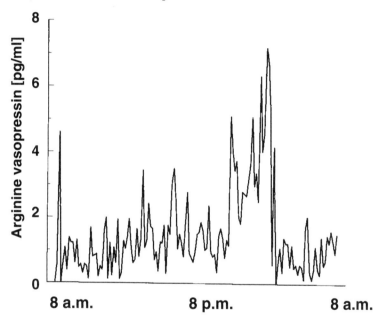

Figure 2–1.   Pattern of plasma arginine vasopressin secretion from a 49-year-old schizophrenic man with polydipsia-hyponatremia syndrome. Blood samples were drawn every 10 minutes for 24 hours. Plasma sodium concentration for the patient ranged between 125 and 133 mmol/L with most values close to 130 mmol/L. During the study, he excreted 24.8 L of urine. There were 24 secretory bursts during the 24-hour study period. The mean ± SD mass of vasopressin secreted per burst was 2.0 ± 0.6 pg/ml. The mean ± SD interburst interval was 58 ± 23 minutes. The mean ± SD maximal rate of vasopressin secretion was 0.19 ± .02 pg/ml per minute. The daily vasopressin secretory rate was 126 pg/ml. Compared with a control subject, the mass of vasopressin secreted per burst, but not the number of vasopressin release episodes, was reduced in this patient with schizophrenia and severe water imbalance.

PULSATILE PATTERNS OF VASOPRESSIN RELEASE

Many endocrine glands secrete their hormones in bursts (Veldhuis and Johnson 1990; Veldhuis et al. 1987; Vieweg et al. 1992b). Frequent venous sampling analysis can identify statistically significant serum or plasma hormone concentration clusters. This clustering is consistent with pulsatile hormone release. The frequency and mass of each burst decide the presence and amount of hormone concentration. An analogy to remember is how firefighters delivered water during the fire brigade era. To bring more water to the fire, they could pass buckets more frequently, pass bigger buckets, or pass bigger buckets more frequently. The posterior lobe of the pituitary gland secretes arginine vasopressin in a pulsatile pattern.

A preliminary report (Vieweg et al. 1991b), subsequently expanded (unpublished data by Vieweg) to include five schizophrenic patients with polydipsia-hyponatremia syndrome and five control subjects, showed that the *mass* of vasopressin secreted per burst, but not the number of vasopressin release episodes, was reduced for schizophrenic patients with polydipsia-hyponatremia syndrome compared with control subjects. Burst mass, not burst frequency, may distinguish schizophrenic patients from control subjects. Water-loaded schizophrenic patients may not be able to sufficiently reduce the mass of vasopressin released with each burst. An antidiuretic state persists in the face of dilutional hyponatremia.

Figure 2–1 shows the pulsatile pattern of vasopressin release in the patient reported by Vieweg et al. (1991b). Note the variability throughout the day with increasing vasopressin values at night. The clinician may misinterpret the meaning of a single vasopressin determination. Graphing frequent venous sampling data shows more clearly the pattern of vasopressin release from the pituitary gland.

Chapter 3

Physiology of Thirst

Sebastian P. Grossman, Ph.D.

L ife evolved in the oceans. As animals ventured onto dry land, they evolved means of storing saline solutions inside their bodies. Humans consist of approximately 60% water (more in young people, less in elderly people). Two-thirds of the total is contained in cells; the remainder constitutes the extracellular fluid that makes up the interstitial fluid immediately surrounding cells and blood plasma confined to the vascular system. The cellular and extracellular fluid compartments are separated by the semipermeable membrane of cells that obstructs the passage of many solutes. The vascular system is separated from interstitial fluid by the walls of blood vessels that are permeable to all but the large protein molecules that are prevalent in blood but not in interstitial fluid. Although the total concentrations of solutes in the two major fluid compartments are equal under normal conditions of hydration (i.e., they are *isotonic*), the nature of the principal electrolytes or their concentrations are quite different. Sodium and chloride are in plentiful supply in the extracellular fluid but present only in small quantity inside cells that, in turn, are rich in potassium, phosphate, and protein.

FLUID COMPARTMENTS

Water and certain salts are essential for survival. Unlike energy, which can be stored in great quantities (mostly in the form of fat), water and salts must be replenished frequently. The human body contains large quantities of water but has little tolerance for even minor decreases in total fluid volume or the concentration of electrolytes contained in it. Yet the human body constantly loses fluids (mostly through evaporation from the skin and lungs, waste product elimination by urine and feces, and sweat that is essential for temperature regulation). This *obligatory fluid loss* amounts to about 2.5 L per day in adult humans. Water and electrolytes (mainly sodium chloride) must be promptly replenished to prevent kidney failure and collapse of the circulatory system.

Water constantly diffuses through cell membranes, but the direction of diffusion is random; hence, there is no net movement into or out of cells. Cells gain or lose water with respect to the extracellular fluid only when the concentration of solutes that do not cross the cell membrane differs between the cellular and extracellular fluids. When a semipermeable membrane that is impermeable to the solutes but permeable to the solvent separates solutions of unequal concentrations of solutes, the solvent moves, by a process of osmosis, into the region of higher concentration until the concentrations of both solutions is equal. Osmotic pressure is determined by the number of molecules or ions in a solution and this *molar concentration* is measured in *osmoles*. One osmole equals the number of particles in 1 g molecular weight of undissociated solute. Osmolality refers to the number of osmoles per kilogram of water. The osmolality of plasma in normally hydrated humans is approximately 290 mOsm/kg.

Water and solutes (except most proteins) diffuse freely across capillary walls. In addition, there are several forces that maintain an equilibrium between blood and interstitial fluid. The pumping action of the heart results in capillary pressure that is greater at the arterial side of the capillary bed than at the venous end. The movement of water out of capillaries is further promoted by the oncotic pressure of proteins in the interstitial fluids and by the fact that its pressure is slightly less than atmospheric pressure. The oncotic pressure of blood proteins opposes the movement of fluid out of the vascular bed, leaving a net outward force of about 13 mm Hg in humans. The oncotic pressure of blood proteins (and the associated positive ions) is also the principal force that returns water to the capillaries. It is opposed by (relatively weak) capillary pressure at the venous end of the capillary bed and by the negative pressure and oncotic pressure of the interstitial fluid. This system of opposing forces results in a small net gain of the interstitial fluid. Equilibrium is reestablished by the movement of water and protein into the lymphatic system that returns the excess to the vascular bed.

Water deprivation results in profound systemic changes in the distribution of body fluids. As water and electrolytes are lost from the circulation, its osmolality rises. This increase results in osmotic concentration gradients that cause the movement of water out of cells and into the extracellular fluid compartment. This action counteracts the volume depletion of the vascular bed and prevents hypotension. It also results in cellular dehydration that activates osmoreceptors in the brain, which initiate a cascade of hormonal and neural events that promote fluid and electrolyte retention by the kidney and give rise to the sensation of thirst. Unless water is readily available, this *osmoregulatory* mechanism is increasingly unable to supply sufficient water to the extracellular compartment and a second, *volumetric,* mechanism eventually comes into play. As the volume (and pressure) of blood falls, a second cascade of neural and hormonal mechanisms is activated, which activates additional brain mechanisms as well as peripheral neural pathways to conserve electrolytes and body fluids and stimulate thirst.

In humans and most other mammals, two regulatory mechanisms have evolved to guarantee adequate hydration and salt concentration. As the body loses fluids and salt, the kidney begins to excrete smaller and smaller amounts of increasingly concentrated urine, thus conserving scarce resources. The sensation of thirst ensures the replenishment of fluids as soon as water becomes available. Because the obligatory loss of body fluids also depletes solutes (mainly sodium chloride), some species develop a specific salt appetite that leads to the preferential ingestion of sodium chloride. Others, including humans, obtain sufficient salt in their diet and rarely experience a conscious need for salt.

HORMONAL MECHANISMS OF CONSERVATION

Arginine Vasopressin

Water deprivation decreases extracellular fluid volume and increases its osmolality. A less than 1% rise (to 292 mOsm/kg) is sufficient to increase the secretion from the posterior pituitary gland of arginine vasopressin (AVP), which acts on the distal tubules of the kidney to cause the retention of water (Robertson et al. 1976). When water deprivation continues, AVP release continues to rise in parallel with plasma osmolality. AVP is also released by a decrease in blood volume, but hypovolemia is an effective stimulus only after the decrease in volume has exceeded 10%–15% of normal levels (Dunn et al. 1973, Fitzsimons 1961b). Hypervolemia raises the osmotic threshold for AVP release (Quillen and Cowley 1983). During prolonged water deprivation, hypovolemia lowers the osmotic threshold for AVP release (McKinley 1985).

When humans are normally hydrated, sufficient AVP is released to permit the use of approximately 50% of the kidney's capacity to retain water. Maximal urine concentration occurs at approximately 294 mOsm/kg. Excessive fluid intake increases plasma volume and decreases its osmolality and AVP release ceases, causing the excretion of maximally dilute urine. Humans begin to experience thirst when blood osmolality reaches approximately 294 mOsm/kg (Baylis and Robertson 1985; Robertson and Athar 1976; Robertson et al. 1976).

Arginine vasopressin is synthesized by magnocellular neurosecretory cells in the *supraoptic nuclei* and *paraventricular nuclei* of the hypothalamus. Projections from these nuclei carry AVP via the *median eminence* to the posterior pituitary where it is stored (Swanson and Sawchenko 1983) and released in response to fluid deficits (Weindl and Sofroniew 1985). When these projections are transected, polyuria and polydipsia occur (R. W. Smith and McCann 1964). The activity of the neurosecretory cells of the supraoptic nuclei and paraventricular nuclei is affected by changes in the osmolality of plasma (Brimble and Dyball 1977) and correlates highly with AVP release (Wakerly and Lincoln 1971). The cells do not appear to be osmosensitive (Haller and Wakerly 1980) but respond to inputs from osmoreceptors in other portions of the preoptic region such as the tissues surrounding the anteroventral third ventricle (AV3V) (Swanson and Sawchenko 1980).

The modulating influences of blood volume changes on AVP release are mediated both neurally and hormonally. The neural input arises from stretch receptors in the right atrium of the heart and adjacent portions of the vena cava and from baroreceptors in the left atrium and adjacent regions of the pulmonary vein (McKinley, 1985; Share 1988). The information is transmitted via the vagus and glossopharyngeal nerves to neurons in the nucleus of the solitary tract, which, in turn, project directly and/or indirectly to the supraoptic nuclei, paraventricular nuclei, and anteromedial preoptic region (Norgren 1981). The hormonal response to hypovolemia consists of the release of renin from the kidney; the renin is converted to angiotensin (the active principle is angiotensin-II [A-II] or angiotensin-III [A-III] in some species). Systemic infusions of angiotensin have been shown to increase AVP release, presumably because of a direct action on the subfornial organ, which projects to the AV3V (Shade and Share 1975; Turker 1986).

Aldosterone

The principal electrolyte in all body fluids, sodium, is as closely regulated as water itself because it is essential for cellular metabolism as well as for the maintenance of blood pressure, volume, and osmolality. Sodium is lost from skin, kidney, salivary glands, and gastrointestinal tract. When plasma sodium levels fall, the vascular system becomes hypovolemic and the kidney releases renin that is converted into A-II. In turn, A-II increases the synthesis and release of aldosterone from the adrenal cortex (Spielman and Davis 1974). Aldosterone reduces sodium excretion in urine, saliva, and perspiration (Ganong 1971). In rats, aldosterone, acting synergistically with angiotensin, elicits a specific salt appetite (Fluharty and Epstein 1983). Adrenalectomy causes an uncontrolled loss of sodium from the kidney as well as salivary and sweat glands and the colon (Richter 1936).

SYSTEMIC ASPECTS OF THIRST

Well into the 20th century, physiologists and psychologists believed that the sensation of thirst was the result of a dry mouth. However, experimental treatments that abolish salivation (e.g., drugs and surgical removal of salivary glands) were shown to increase the frequency of drinking but not the total amount of fluid ingested. A dry mouth does accompany thirst, but wetting the mouth does not relieve thirst. More recent experiments have shown that humans can distinguish between the sensations that arise after water deprivation and those related to a dry mouth alone (Rolls et al. 1980b). The contemporary interpretation of thirst is that it is a sensation of general origin that cannot be attributed to any particular sensory organ.

Humans and many animals drink in excess of physiological need when water or other palatable fluids are available. Much of this "secondary" drinking occurs during meals. In humans, taste, social pressures, and central nervous system effects, rather than true thirst, are major factors in the consumption of fluids such as coffee, tea, or alcoholic beverages (Rolls et al. 1978).

Behavioral Observations

When water or other fluids are available ad libitum, humans as well as many mammals drink mainly in association with meals and ingest more fluid than needed to replenish normal body water stores. In such circumstances the body becomes a "kidney regulator," ingesting more water (as well as sodium in the diet) than necessary and regulating body fluid volume and composition largely by excretion.

In more natural situations where water is available only intermittently, and is often a scare commodity, the relation of drinking to physiological need is monitored more closely. Many species such as dogs, sheep, and deer begin to drink as soon as water becomes available and continue to drink until the amount ingested is just about equal to the existing fluid deficit. Others, such as humans, guinea pigs, and rats, stop after replacing 50%–75% of their fluid deficit and drink intermittently thereafter until actual needs are met (Adolph 1943; Adoph 1964).

Most species that compensate promptly for the existing water deficit stop long before the ingested water can restore the cellular and extracellular fluid deficits. The volume of the ingested fluid appears to be "metered" orally or gastrically. Dogs, for instance, drink enough in 2–3 minutes to fully compensate for the deficit incurred as a result of a 24-hour fast, yet significant changes in the volume and concentration of plasma do not occur until

10–12 minutes after the onset of drinking (Rolls et al. 1980a) and the complete restoration of predeprivation fluid levels occurs only after 45–60 minutes (Ramsay et al. 1977). In humans, drinking slows significantly as much as 10 minutes before changes in plasma sodium (and cellular hydration) occur (Rolls et al. 1980a, 1980b).

Physiological Mechanisms

Oral sensations are not essential for the experience of thirst as we have seen earlier. However, they do play a significant role in the regulation of water intake, as numerous experiments on animals with esophageal, gastric, or duodenal fistulae have shown. Sham drinking occurs in animals with esophageal, gastric, or duodenal fistulae. Water wets the mouth but exits the body before reaching the stomach.

Esophageal fistulae. Claude Bernard reported nearly 150 years ago that many mammals with esophageal fistulae sham drink large amounts of water that are far in excess of actual need (Bernard 1856). Modern investigations have shown, however, that sham drinking is, in fact, proportional to the existing fluid needs. Some species such as sheep, goats, and camels are so good at "oral metering" that they stop for a longer rest after sham drinking a quantity of water that would satisfy physiological needs were it allowed to be absorbed (Adoph 1964; Schmidt-Nielsen et al. 1956). Others overdrink extensively, but total intake remains proportional to actual fluid deficits (Blass and Hall 1976).

These experiments clearly indicate that wetting the mouth of a thirsty subject provides sufficient incentive to drink, but they also demonstrate that wetting the mouth does not provide true satiety. The proportionality between intake and actual fluid deficit indicates the efficacy of oral metering. The mechanisms for oral metering are as yet poorly understood, although oral water or saline receptors, which project to the anteromedial preoptic region, have been implicated (Liljestrand and Zotterman 1954).

Intragastric infusions. Intubation of water into the stomach of water-deprived animals reduces subsequent oral drinking. The magnitude of the effect varies among species. When enough water is infused to distend the stomach, many species do not drink at all. These effects presumably are mediated by stretch receptors because the inflation of stomach balloons (N. E. Miller et al. 1957) or tests conducted before a significant amount of water could be absorbed (Adolph 1950; O'Kelly et al. 1954) produced similar effects.

When water is slowly instilled via permanently indwelling gastric fistulae at a rate calculated to approximate the rate of normal drinking, subsequent oral intake is reduced by about 0.4 ml for each milliliter infused intragastrically (Fitzsimons 1971b). Discrete intragastric infusions of water just before and during each meal reduced oral water intake by about 0.3 ml for each 1 ml infused (Nicolaidis and Rowland 1975, Rowland and Nicolaidis 1976).

Removal of fluid from stomach or duodenum. A series of experiments that has significantly contributed to our understanding of gastric and duodenal satiety influences involved draining orally ingested fluid from the gastrointestinal tract (Maddison et al. 1980; Wood et al. 1980). When orally ingested water is drained via a stomach fistula, monkeys drink almost immediately and replace most of the drained fluid. When deprived monkeys are permitted to drink water while the gastric fistula is open, they consume five to six times the amount consumed while the fistula is closed.

A second group of experiments involved drainage of orally ingested water from the stomach while water or isotonic saline was intubated into the duodenum. Isotonic saline failed to reduce sham drinking, whereas water reduced it by approximately 50%. On balance, these experiments indicate that in the monkey the presence of water in the stomach is a major factor in preabsorptive satiety, whereas oral factors appear to be of little consequence. The absorption of water from the duodenum produces partial satiety even when orally ingested water is drained from the stomach, even when the duodenal infusion is larger than the amount that would normally enter the duodenum from the stomach at the time of testing.

Intravenous injections of water. When water is infused intravenously in the monkey, sham drinking is not reduced (Wood et al. 1980), even though plasma sodium concentrations fall to levels below those produced by intraduodenal infusions. These results suggest that the absorption of water from the duodenum activates satiety sensors that are not sensitive to plasma dilution. The existence of satiety-related hepatic osmoreceptors has been postulated, but the empirical evidence for hepatic satiety mechanisms is, as yet, limited (Kozlowski and Drzewiecki 1973).

Experiments with rats have indicated that the pattern of intragastric and intravenous infusions affects their efficacy greatly (Nicolaidis and Rowland 1975; Rowland and Nicolaidis 1976). Continuous intragastric infusions are far more satiating than intravenous infusions. However, discrete intravenous injections during ad libitum meals are more effective than similarly spaced intragastric injections. Discrete intravenous and intragastric injections, administered during the interval between meals, are equally effective. The importance of postabsorptive satiety signals has been further demonstrated in experiments showing that rats can be trained to regulate their fluid balance by self-administering discrete intravenous injections of water (Nicolaidis and Rowland 1974).

CELLULAR AND EXTRACELLULAR INFLUENCES ON THIRST

Water deprivation initially reduces the volume and osmolality of extracellular fluids (blood plasma and interstitial fluids). The resulting osmotic forces cause water to be drawn out of cells. Cellular dehydration is thus the first signal for thirst. If deprivation persists, the cells cannot give up enough water to maintain blood volume. The resulting hypovolemia is the second thirst signal, which coexists, under normal circumstances, with cellular dehydration. Animal experiments have shown that systemic injections of water (that reverse cellular dehydration but have no lasting effects on blood volume) reduce drinking after a fast by 65%–85%. Similar injections of isotonic saline (which replenish plasma volume but do not affect cellular hydration) reduce drinking by only 5%–25% (Ramsay and Thrasher 1986; Wood et al. 1982). Thus, cellular dehydration is by far the more important stimulus for thirst, at least for relatively brief periods of deprivation. Hypovolemic thirst may indeed be mainly a mechanism for dealing with emergencies such as a sudden loss of blood or severe diarrhea.

The importance of osmotic mechanisms in the regulation of thirst and body water regulation has been demonstrated in experiments showing that systemic injections of hypertonic solutions containing solutes such as sodium chloride that cannot cross the semipermeable cell membrane elicit drinking as well as AVP release. Similarly, hypertonic solutions containing solutes, such as glucose, that can freely enter cells have no effect. Because the kidney can excrete a significant amount of the added solutes, the effect of hypertonic saline is often quite variable except in nephrectomized animals (Fitzsimons 1961a).

In the rat, the cellular-dehydration thirst signals appear to originate mainly in "osmoreceptors" located in the lateral preoptic region and the tissues surrounding the AV3V. Microinjections of hypertonic saline into these areas elicit drinking in sated animals (Blass and Epstein 1971; Buggy 1977) and alter the neural activity of cells in the region (Nicolaidis and Jeulin 1984). Microinjections of water into the lateral preoptic region selectively reduce the drinking response to systemic injections of hypertonic saline (Blass and Epstein 1971). Systemic injections of hypertonic saline also modify the activity of cells in the area (Blank and Wayner 1975). Some lesions in the preoptic area (Blass and Epstein 1971) selectively reduce or abolish the drinking response to systemic injections of hypertonic saline. Damage to the AV3V has similar effects on cellular thirst but also reduces the drinking response to some extracellular stimuli (Buggy and Johnson 1977a).

Although contemporary interest has concentrated on these regions, lesions in other areas of the brain (e.g., the zona incerta) selectively abolish drinking responses to systemic hypertonic saline (S. P. Grossman and Grossman 1978). Osmoreceptors have also been found in the hepatic portal system. These cells communicate with neurons in the hypothalamus (Smitt 1973), and there is some evidence suggesting that they may influence water intake in the rat (Kraly 1978) and dog (Kozlowski and Drzewiecki 1973).

In some species such as the goat, specialized sodium receptors may take the place of osmoreceptors. Intracerebroventricular injections of hypertonic sodium chloride solutions elicit drinking and

AVP release in this species, whereas equally hyperosmotic solutions of sucrose, fructose, or mannitol, which are also excluded from transport into cells, do not (Andersson 1978). Sheep may have both osmoreceptors and sodium receptors. In this species intracerebroventricular injections of sucrose do elicit drinking when dissolved in artificial cerebrospinal fluid (this avoids the sodium depletion seen when water is used as the solvent), but the effect is smaller than that of similarly hypertonic injections of sodium chloride (McKinley et al. 1978).

Extracellular Dehydration (Hypovolemic) Thirst

Hemorrhage. Physicians staffing emergency departments have long known that patients with severe diarrhea or blood loss complain of intense thirst (Fitzsimons 1979). Experimental investigations of this phenomenon have shown that a blood loss of 10%–15% results in drinking, decreased urine flow, and a delayed salt appetite in the rat (Fitzsimons 1961b). Thirst and renal water conservation cannot, in this case, be caused by cellular dehydration because the loss of isotonic plasma does not alter the osmotic pressure of extracellular fluids. Unlike many other forms of extracellular thirst stimuli, the efficacy of hemorrhage is not angiotensin dependent (Fitzsimons 1961b). The amount of fluid ingested is directly proportional to the blood loss over a wide range (Russell et al. 1975).

Hypernatremia. Early clinical observations also documented elevated thirst after sodium chloride deprivation (which dilutes extracellular fluid and thereby causes cellular overhydration and extracellular hypovolemia) (Strauss 1957). In the rat, salt-deficient diets increase water intake (Radford 1959). Intraperitoneal glucose dialysis has similar effects. In these experiments, intraperitoneal injections of isotonic glucose are allowed to equilibrate with extracellular fluid before an equal amount of fluid, containing sodium chloride and other electrolytes, is withdrawn. This rapid removal of sodium chloride results in the movement of water into cells and thus results in hypovolemia (Falk and Tang 1980).

Experimental edema. Most of the hundreds of investigations of the effects of extracellular hypovolemia have used intraperitoneal (Fitzsimons 1961b) or subcutaneous (Stricker 1966) injections of hyperoncotic concentrations of polyethylene glycol. This colloid disrupts the Starling equilibrium of capillaries and withdraws isotonic, protein-free plasma from the circulation and sequesters it in an edema at the injection site. Because the osmolality of the extracellular fluid is not changed, cellular hydration is not affected. Rats begin to drink 1–2 hours after polyethylene glycol treatment and conserve water as well as sodium, at least in part, in response to increased secretion of AVP (Dunn et al. 1973), aldosterone, and renin (Stricker et al. 1979). Drinking stops 8–10 hours after the polyethylene glycol treatment, presumably because of osmotic dilution. (Cellular overhydration has been eliminated as a potential candidate for satiety [Stricker 1981].)

When both water and hypertonic saline are available, rats drink mostly water during the first 6 hours after polyethylene glycol, even though water alone cannot remedy the vascular hypovolemia. They then begin to drink saline and alternate between saline and water for the next 12–18 hours. The total fluid ingested remains slightly hypotonic (Stricker 1981). The sodium ingested during this period is largely retained and the vascular hyponatremia is reversed. This effect draws water out of the cells and completes the restoration of the extracellular fluid volume.

When water and saline are withheld during the first 8 hours after polyethylene glycol, rats initially drink only water. They eventually do switch to the pattern of alternating saline and water intake, but the initial bout of water ingestion indicates that the thirst elicited by activation of the renin-angiotensin mechanisms (below) supersedes the salt appetite that is well established at this point. When water and saline are withheld for 24 hours after polyethylene glycol ingestion, rats immediately display the alternation pattern, and the mixture produces a total fluid intake that is the isotonic fluid necessary to restore a normal fluid balance

Caval ligation. Several procedures have been used to demonstrate that extracellular thirst may not be a result of a decrease in blood volume per se but, instead, a result of a decrease in blood pressure.

Ligation of the inferior vena cava, which carries approximately 30% of the venous return to the heart, lowers arterial blood pressure and elicits drinking in the rat. Urine volume and urine sodium and potassium excretion are severely reduced (Fitzsimons 1964). The effect is markedly diminished by nephrectomy, indicating that the renin-angiotensin system may play a significant role in caval ligation-induced thirst. This conclusion is supported by the observation that constriction of the renal arteries results in the same syndrome as ligation of the inferior vena cava (Fitzsimons 1969).

Hormonal Influences on Thirst

The renin-angiotensin system.   Extracellular thirst stimuli result in hypovolemia and hypotension. This result, in turn, modulates the activity of baro- or stretch receptors in the great veins and low pressure chambers of the heart, which communicate with the brain stem via the vagus and the sympathetic afferents. This neural pathway is important for brain mechanisms concerned with thirst and AVP release.

Hypovolemia and hypotension also activate the renin-angiotensin system that provides a second, nonneural signal to brain mechanisms related to thirst and to AVP release. As we have seen in our brief review of some of the clinical conditions and experimental procedures that result in hypovolemic thirst, the role of angiotensin has been the subject of some controversy. Under some conditions, it appears to be an essential component of the message to the brain that water needs to be conserved and replenished; under others, it seems to provide mainly an early warning signal.

Angiotensin and related receptor mechanisms have been found in many areas of the brain, and it has been suggested (Ganong 1984) that there may be separate brain angiotensin systems where the hormone may act as a neurotransmitter or neuromodulator. This interpretation is supported by the fact that angiotensin is a large peptide that cannot cross the blood-brain barrier. It can enter the brain at certain circumventricular organs where the blood-brain barrier is absent or weak, but this does not account for its widespread distribution in the central nervous system.

Yet, A-II (and, in some species, its breakdown product A-III) is an extremely potent dipsogen in nearly all species tested to date, including mammals, birds, and such esoteric laboratory animals as eels, iguana, and euryhaline killifish. Systemic injections are not effective in a few species such as gerbils, goats, and sheep. However, these apparent exceptions to the rule do drink in response to intracranial injections of very small quantities of angiotensin. For a detailed review of the variety of angiotensin-sensitive species, see Fitzsimons (1979). Some, but not all, humans drink in response to systemic angiotensin, and there is no difference between drinkers and nondrinkers in plasma angiotensin levels (Rolls et al. 1986). The effects of angiotensin are behaviorally specific to thirst and thirst-related behaviors (McFarland and Rolls 1972; Rolls et al. 1972).

Many of the seminal experiments in this field are based on doses of angiotensin that are in excess of those found in plasma after 24 or 48 hours of water deprivation. It has therefore been argued that angiotensin might play merely a "permissive" role in extracellular drinking by elevating blood pressure to the point where the test animal can make appropriate drinking or water-seeking responses to extracellular dehydration (Stricker 1978). However, more accurate radioimmunoassay measures of A-II plasma levels have indicated, more recently, that dipsogenic doses of angiotensin produce lower plasma levels of A-II than 14 or 48 hours of water deprivation or various experimental procedures that reliably induced extracellular thirst (Johnson et al. 1986; Mann et al. 1980).

A number of investigators have attempted to elucidate the role of angiotensin in thirst by blocking its synthesis—or receptor—action pharmacologically. The most commonly used receptor blocker is saralasin (or P113). Systemic injections of this compound have been reported to inhibit drinking as a response to intravenous renin or A-II without impairing drinking responses to hypertonic saline or some extracellular thirst stimuli such as various hypotensive agents (Tang and Falk 1974). Intracranial injections of minute quantities of saralasin block the drinking responses to systemic as well as intracranial A-II (Felix et al. 1986) without reducing the response to systemic hypertonic saline or water deprivation (M. C. Lee et al. 1981; Summy-Long and Severs 1974).

The early literature on the systemic or central effects of inhibitors of the converting enzyme responsible for the transformation of the inactive form angiotensin I (A-I) to the dipsogenic form A-II used a weak agent code named SQ 20881. These investigations produced some unexpected results, including facilitatory effects on drinking responses to isoproterenol (discussed below), caval ligation, polyethylene-induced hypoglycemia, or water deprivation, after systemic injections of SQ 20881 (Lehr et al. 1973, 1975). Intracranial injections inhibited drinking in response to renin as expected but had no effect on drinking in response to isoproterenol or caval ligation (Lehr et al. 1973, 1975).

More recent investigations have used captopril, a more powerful converting enzyme inhibitor (see de Caro, Epstein, and Massi 1986 for review). Low systemic doses of captopril have facilitatory effects on various extracellular dipsogen and even elicit some drinking (Lehr et al. 1973). Intracranial injections of captopril inhibit drinking and sodium intake in response to intracerebroventricular injections of A-I but not to A-II (Weiss 1986).

The apparently paradoxical facilitatory effects of systemic SQ 2088 and captopril may result from the fact that the converting enzyme inhibitors do not cross the blood-brain barrier unless administered in high doses. The lack of A-I to A-II conversion increases the amount of A-I (not only because the lack of conversion increases the short-term availability of A-I, but also because the scarcity of A-II removes an inhibitory feedback on renin-secreting mechanisms in the kidney). The increase in plasma levels of A-I promotes its uptake into the brain where it can be converted to A-II. The model is supported by the fact that high systemic doses of captopril, which permit the entry of significant amounts of converting enzyme inhibitor into the brain, reduce drinking in response to polyethylene glycol (Ramsay and Thrasher 1986).

β-Adrenergic thirst.   Drugs such as isoproterenol decrease blood pressure by a direct action on smooth muscle. They also act directly on renal receptors, and the two effects combine to release large quantities of renin (Ganong 1972). In the rat, the result is copious drinking and antidiuresis (Lehr et al. 1967). Some species, such as goats, that do not drink in response to angiotensin also fail to drink after isoproterenol treatments (K. Olson and Rundgren 1975). β-Adrenergic antagonists such as propranolol block the dipsogenic and renin-releasing activity of isoproterenol in the rat (Lehr et al. 1967; Meyer et al. 1971).

The putative role of the renin-angiotensin system in β-adrenergic thirst has been the subject of controversy. Several investigators have reported that nephrectomy abolishes the drinking response to isoproterenol, for example (Meyer et al. 1971), but more recent investigations have indicated that the inhibition may be only partial (Ramsay and Thrasher 1986). Nephrectomized rats that did not drink in response to isoproterenol did so when blood pressure was elevated by pressure agents such as epinephrine (Hosutt et al. 1978). This response may indicate that the nephrectomized rat is unable to deal with the stress of hypotension and fails to drink because of general behavioral incompetence. It has also been suggested that nephrectomy abolishes the drinking response to low doses of isoproterenol, which release renin but have only minor effects on blood pressure. The response to higher doses, which produce severe hypotension, in contrast, may be able to affect extrarenal neural pathways to activate brain mechanisms related to thirst and AVP secretion (Ramsay and Thrasher 1986).

Pharmacological investigations have had mixed success in relating isoproterenol drinking to the renin-angiotensin system. Systemic infusions of the competitive angiotensin-receptor blocker *saralasin*, which blocks the drinking response to angiotensin, have been reported not to reduce the drinking response to various hypotensive agents, including isoproterenol (Tang and Falk 1974). Saralasin does inhibit β-adrenergic drinking when administered intracranially (Schwob and Johnson 1975). The two results are not contradictory because saralasin does not readily cross the blood-brain barrier. Together, the two observations suggest that β-adrenergic drinking may be related to a central action of angiotensin. Matters are complicated, however, by the observation that SQ 20881, a drug that inhibits the conversion of inactive A-I to the dipsogenic A-II, paradoxically facilitates isoproterenol drinking when administered systemically (Lehr et al. 1973). It has no effect on the drinking response to isoproterenol when administered intracerebroventricularly, even though the same intracerebro-ventricular injections inhibit A-II-induced drinking (Lehr et al. 1973). We shall return to the thorny issues surrounding the role of the renin-angiotensin system in thirst shortly.

Atrial natriuretic factor. The pioneering research of de Bold and associates first demonstrated that injections of extracts of rat myocardial atrial tissue result in pronounced natriuresis and diuresis (A. J. de Bold et al. 1981). Despite more than a decade of intensive research, we have, as yet, only a sketchy picture of the role of the active principle in this extract, the polypeptide hormone natriuretic factor or atriopeptin, in the regulation of blood pressure and extracellular thirst. The hormone exerts a potent natriuretic and diuretic effect; produces regional vaso relaxation; and inhibits renin, aldosterone, and vasopressin release (A. J. de Bold 1986).

Extracts from water-deprived (Johnson et al. 1986) or salt-loaded (Ackerman and Irizawa 1984) rats have elevated atriopeptin activity. More specifically, water deprivation increases cardiac atrio-peptin stores while decreasing the amount in plasma (Takayanagi et al. 1985). When water-deprived rats are salt loaded, the cardiac stores of atriopeptin decrease and plasma levels increase (Takayanagi et al. 1985). Similarly, rats maintained on a high-salt diet have low cardiac stores of atriopeptin, whereas rats maintained on a low-salt diet have elevated levels (Manning et al. 1985). Hypervolemia releases atriopeptin and results in natriuresis and diuresis. The renal response to hypervolemia is greatly attenuated when the source of atriopeptin (the right atrium of the heart) is removed (Veress and Sonnenberg 1984). Lastly, there is evidence that vasopressin releases atriopeptin, although pharmacological doses were used to demonstrate this effect (Manning et al. 1985).

The role of atriopeptin in thirst and extracellular fluid regulation has been controversial. Some investigators (Blaine 1986) believe that it plays a major role as a "counterbalance" to the renin-angiotensin system. Others (Gellai et al. 1986) suggest that it may play only a local role in modulating the sensitivity of atrial stretch receptors. According to this view, hormonal effects on distant organs such as the kidney and adrenal gland might be caused by the use of nonphysiological experimental conditions.

BRAIN MECHANISMS OF THIRST

Anatomical Studies

Lateral and medial hypothalamus.   Bilateral lesions in the lateral hypothalamus result in adipsia, usually accompanied by aphagia (Anand and Brobeck 1951). Voluntary ingestive behavior gradually recovers after weeks or even months of total fasting (Teitelbaum and Epstein 1962). The animals that have "recovered" from lateral hypothalamus lesions drink amounts of water that are commensurate with their permanently decreased body weight. They do not drink when food deprived, suggesting that water intake is motivated not by thirst but by a need to facilitate chewing and swallowing food (Epstein and Teitelbaum 1964). This hypothesis is supported by the observation that recovered animals are purely prandial drinkers (i.e., they drink after each bite of dry food rather than before and after a meal) (Kissileff 1969, Kissileff and Epstein 1969).

Also in agreement with this notion is the consistent finding that the animal that has recovered from lateral hypothalamus lesions responds poorly if at all to experimental treatments (discussed above) that give rise to cellular or extracellular dehydration and, in normal animals, elicit drinking (Epstein and Teitelbaum 1964).

The observed impairments appear to be specifically related to thirst. The animals are not oblivious to their salt and water needs. When injected with hypertonic saline, they excrete much of the salt in highly concentrated urine. Only when this mechanism appears to be exhausted does a little drinking occur after a delay of many hours (Stricker 1976).

The conclusion that lateral hypothalamus lesions damage a neural system specifically related to thirst has been challenged on the basis of observations indicating severe sensory motor and arousal dysfunctions following lateral hypothalamus lesions. These are mainly a result of an interruption of dopaminergic *nigrostriatal projections* that pass through the lateral hypothalamus. The severe sensory motor and arousal dysfunctions recover in parallel with ingestive behavior (Balagura et al. 1969).

Lesions elsewhere (e.g., the substantia nigra [Marshall et al. 1974] and globus pallidus [Morgane 1961]) as well as knife cuts that sever the nigrostriatal projections without damage to cellular components of the lateral hypothalamus (Alheid et al. 1977) produce similar effects on sensory motor functions and ingestive behavior.

There can be little doubt that the sensory motor and arousal deficits seen in rats with lateral hypothalamus lesions contribute to and may be fully responsible for the aphagia and adipsia seen during the immediate postoperative period. Several observations indicate, however, that neural mechanisms specifically related to thirst also are destroyed by the lesion. The recovered lateral animal is fully capable of drinking in response to prandial and, perhaps, digestive needs, yet it does not drink when deprived of food and does not correct fluid deficits incurred during water deprivation unless food is also available. It also fails to drink to experimental treatments that induce cellular or extracellular dehydration (see the discussion above). To suggest that these "residual deficits" may reflect subclinical impairments in sensory, motor, or arousal functions as some investigators have suggested (Stricker 1976) would seem to stretch one's imagination a bit far. Although these animals do not drink water in response to hypertonic saline treatments, they avidly drink milk (a preferred liquid), suggesting that they are quite capable of drinking at a time when there appears to be insufficient motivation to ingest plain water (D. R. Williams and Teitelbaum 1959).

Transient adipsia and impaired drinking to osmotic challenges also have been reported after microinjections of the neurotoxin kainic acid, which destroyed nerve cell bodies in the lateral hypothalamus without affecting fibers of passage (Grossman et al. 1978; Stricker et al. 1978). The kainic-acid-treated animals showed no evidence of sensory motor or arousal impairments and were indeed hyperactive and hyperreactive to somatic stimuli (Grossman et al. 1978).

There are reports indicating that cellular and extracellular thirst may be affected differentially by different hypothalamic lesions. On the one hand, damage to medial components of the lateral hypothalamus has been reported to impair drinking responses to extracellular thirst stimuli such as renin, angiotensin, or isoproterenol without affecting the drinking response to hypertonic saline

(Sclafani et al. 1973). Lesions in lateral aspects of the lateral hypothalamus, on the other hand, have been reported to produce an
opposite pattern of effects, the drinking response to cellular dehydration being selectively impaired or abolished (Kucharczyk and
Mogenson 1975).

Lesions in the posterior aspects of the ventromedial hypothalamus result in hyperdipsia, often accompanied by hyperphagia
(R. W. Smith and McCann 1964) as well as an apparently selective
hyperreactivity to hypertonic saline (King and Grossman 1977).
Nephrectomy does not abolish the hyperdipsia, suggesting that a
disruption of vasopressin release may not be responsible for the
effect. Knife cuts that transect the posterior connections of the ventromedial hypothalamus also produce hyperdipsia, which is only
partially reversed by large doses of vasopressin (Hennessy et al.
1977). A recent exhaustive study of the effects of knife cuts in the
region indicates that they do affect vasopressin release significantly
(Andrews 1993).

Electrical stimulation of the lateral hypothalamus elicits copious and often sustained drinking that can result in the ingestion of
very large quantities of water (N. E. Miller 1960; Mogenson and
Stevenson 1967). Stimulation of the region also can elicit other behaviors such as eating, gnawing, and so on (N. E. Miller 1960), and
the nature of the response is often determined by environmental
factors (e.g., the presence of food, water, or wooden blocks). Moreover, some animals that initially display only drinking can be induced to switch when only food is available during the stimulation
session (Valenstein et al. 1968). This variability may, of course, result from the fact that the region subserves many basic motivational systems that appear to be closely intertwined anatomically.
Electrical stimulation may thus activate several different systems.
However, some investigators have proposed that the stimulation
may have general arousal properties, thus leading to whatever behavior may be appropriate in a given situation (Valenstein 1973).
Although this fits nicely with the decreased arousal interpretation
of the effects of lateral hypothalamus lesions, considerable evidence
suggests that more specific effects on thirst-related mechanisms
are involved. At some electrode sites, only drinking can be elicited, especially when small electrodes are employed that reduce

the spread of electrical current (Mogenson 1971). Moreover, the current threshold (Wise 1969) and / or stimulation frequency (Mogenson et al. 1971) for eliciting drinking is often different from that required to elicit other behaviors. Electrophysiological studies have identified single cells in the hypothalamus that respond, apparently selectively, to systemic salt loads, salt or water on the tongue (Nicolaidis 1968), or direct iontophoretic applications of sodium to the cell (Oomura et al. 1969). The behavioral evidence for the specificity of stimulation-induced drinking also includes reports that water loads, which reduce deprivation-induced drinking, also increase the threshold for stimulation-induced drinking (Mendelson 1970). Also, hypothalamic stimulation elicits instrumental behaviors previously associated with water rewards (B. Andersson and Wyrwicka 1957).

The zona incerta. Immediately dorsal to the lateral hypothalamus lies the zona incerta, which has been implicated in the regulation of thirst. Lesions in this structure do not produce the sensory motor and arousal dysfunctions seen after lateral hypothalamus lesions (Walsh and Grossman 1973), and electrical stimulation of the area elicits only drinking (Huang and Mogenson 1972). The interpretation of the effects of lesions or stimulation in the region is thus not plagued by the problems encountered in the lateral hypothalamus.

Zona incerta lesions produce transient mild hypodipsia and total adipsia during periods of food deprivation (Walsh and Grossman 1973). The adipsia appears to be permanent (Grossman and Grossman 1978). When food is made available after 24 hours of food deprivation (and no drinking), rats with zona incerta lesions eat a significant amount of food before taking their first drink. They also make no effort to make up the fluid lost during the self-imposed water restriction. When food is present during water deprivation, rats with zona incerta lesions promptly drink a large quantity of water as soon as it is made available, although the total intake is slightly reduced compared with that seen in intact control subjects (Walsh and Grossman 1978). Clearly, the rat with zona incerta lesions is a purely prandial drinker. This conclusion is confirmed by the observation that the rat with zona incerta lesions drinks very little or nothing in response to subcutaneous, intraperitoneal, or intravenous injections of a wide range of doses of hypertonic saline (Grossman and Grossman 1978; Rowland et al. 1979).

The effects of zona incerta lesions are caused by the destruction of neurons indigenous to the region because microinjections of the neurotoxin kainic acid, which destroys nerve cell bodies but not fibers of passage, reproduce the effects of electrolytic lesions (B. Brown and Grossman 1980). The effect of zona incerta lesions on extracellular thirst stimuli is curiously variable. Rats with zona incerta lesions do not drink in response to isoproterenol or systemic or intracranial angiotensin (Rowland et al. 1979; Walsh and Grossman 1976). However, they drink normally, or nearly so, during polyethylene glycol- or formalin-induced vascular hypovolemia (Grossman and Grossman 1978; Walsh and Grossman 1976).

Medial preoptic area and AV3V.   Lesions in the medial preoptic area severely disrupt temperature regulation, and this appears to be the principal cause of the general malaise, adipsia, and aphagia that have been reported. Animals that survive the immediate postoperative period recover normal ad libitum food and water intake but remain chronically hypernatremic and unresponsive to systemic salt loads. They drink normally as a response to polyethylene glycol-induced hypovolemia (S. L. Black 1976). When appropriate measures are taken to prevent the disruption of temperature regulation, the postoperative adipsia and aphagia are prevented, but the persisting hypernatremia and unresponsiveness to hypertonic saline are prominent (McGowan et al. 1988a).

Large lesions in the area that includes the medial preoptic region as well as tissues surrounding the AV3V result in adipsia (Johnson and Buggy 1978) and hypernatremia (Buggy and Johnson 1977b). If the animals survive the initial postoperative period, ad libitum drinking returns to normal. However, they drink little or nothing in response to water deprivation, systemic salt loads, isoproterenol, and systemic or intracranial angiotensin. The drinking response to polyethylene glycol-induced hypovolemia is intact (Buggy and Johnson 1977b; Johnson and Buggy 1978). Except for the initial adipsia and hypernatremia, this pattern of effects is comparable to that seen after zona incerta lesions.

The effects of these large lesions are often attributed to the tissues immediately surrounding the anterior ventral third ventricle. However, a recent experiment has shown that lesions restricted to these tissues do not affect ad libitum water intake, plasma osmolality, or drinking responses to deprivation, hypertonic saline, isoproterenol, or systemic angiotensin. Lesions restricted to the adjacent medial preoptic area also had no effect on ad libitum drinking but resulted in hypernatremia and impaired drinking responses to hypertonic saline (McGowan et al. 1988a).

Microinjections of saline or A-II into the AV3V region and adjacent tissues elicit drinking as well as systemic pressor and antidiuretic responses. The effects of the two compounds are not additive (Buggy 1977).

Lateral preoptic region. A number of investigators have reported severely impaired drinking responses to systemic hypertonic saline in rats and other species with lesions in the lateral preoptic region. In some instances, ad libitum drinking and the response to water deprivation appeared to be normal (Blass and Epstein 1971; Peck and Novin 1971). Rats with lateral preoptic region lesions respond to intraperitonial salt loads mainly by increased excretion of sodium, combined with some delayed drinking. They also drink, apparently normally, in response to intravenous injections of hypertonic saline as well as increased salt in their diet (Coburn and Stricker 1978).

The effects of lesions in the lateral preoptic area on extracellular thirst have been the subject of controversy. Some lesions have been reported to selectively impair cellular dehydration thirst. More commonly, lesions in the lateral preoptic region reduce the response to vascular hypovolemia as well (Blass and Epstein 1971; Coburn and Stricker 1978). There was also a report of impaired drinking after systemic angiotensin or isoproterenol in rats with lateral preoptic region lesions that drank normally in response to hypertonic saline (Peck 1973). A recent study of the effects of iontophoretic applications of kainic acid that depleted a subpopulation of cells in the area suggests that the intensity of the thirst stimulus may be an important determinant of the ability of an animal with lateral preoptic region lesions to respond. In this experiment, rats with partial depletions of neurons in the lateral preoptic region drank normal quantities of water after small salt loads as well as low doses of polyethylene glycol but displayed significant impairments in response to larger doses of sodium chloride or polyethylene glycol (McGowan et al. 1988b).

Drinking after microinjections of hypertonic saline into the lateral preoptic region has been reported in rats (Blass and Epstein 1971) and rabbits (Peck and Novin 1971). However, the number of positive injection sites has been disappointingly small, and the sodium chloride concentrations of the minimally effective injections have been considerably higher than anything normally found in tissue. Long-term infusions of more mildly hypertonic solutions have produced increases in the majority of animals tested, but the magnitude of the effects was quite variable (Andrews et al. 1992).

All of this should be viewed in the context of numerous reports of altered single-cell activity in the lateral preoptic region following systemic injections of hypertonic solutions of sodium chloride or sucrose (Blank and Wayner 1975; Malmo and Malmo 1979).

Organum vasculosum of the lamina terminalis and nucleus medianus.   The tissues anterior to the third ventricle are divided into a ventral region containing the organum vasculosum of the lamina terminalis and the subcommissural portion of the nucleus medianus (not to be confused with the medial preoptic area) and a dorsal region containing the subfornical organ, the nucleus medianus, and ventromedial septum. The entire region has been implicated in the regulation of body water and thirst.

In sheep (McKinley et al. 1982, 1983) and goats (B. Anderson et al. 1975) large lesions involving the organum vasculosum of the lamina terminalis and nucleus medianum result in adipsia (only some animals ever recover voluntary water intake) and extreme hypernatremia. Animals that recover from the adipsia do not drink in response to hypertonic salt loads or systemic angiotensin. In rats, more discrete lesions of the nucleus medianus result in an initial period of adipsia, which is followed by hyperdipsia in some animals. Hyperdipsic as well as normodipsic rats from these experiments do not drink in response to systemic cellular or extracellular dehydration when tested during the day but respond normally at night, suggesting that this region may contain a thirst-related activating system (T. W. Gardiner and Stricker 1985a, 1985b).

Septal area.   Some septal lesions (there is no consensus on exactly where the effective lesions are) produce hyperdipsia in rats and reduce AVP release during cellular dehydration but not during extracellular hypovolemia (Iovino and Steardo 1986). The hyperdipsia itself is specifically caused by a facilitatory effect on extracellular thirst. Rats that are hyperdipsic as a consequence of septal lesions drink more than control subjects in response to polyethylene glycol, caval ligation, renin, angiotensin, or isoproterenol but respond normally to salt loads (Blass and Hanson 1970; Blass et al. 1974). Electrical stimulation of the septal area inhibits drinking in response to cellular as well as extracellular thirst stimuli as well as water deprivation (Moran and Blass 1976).

Angiotensin-sensitive brain mechanisms.   As discussed above, all extracellular thirst stimuli activate the renin-angiotensin system, although it is not yet entirely clear to what extent this contributes to extracellular thirst. Two hypotheses that are not mutually exclusive have been proposed to account for the dipsogenic effects of A-II (Fitzsimons 1969, 1971a).

Angiotensin may modulate the activity of baro- and stretch receptors in the great veins and atria of the heart that are known to send blood pressure-related information to the hypothalamus via vagal afferents. Although plausible, it has been all but impossible to investigate the proposed interaction because all procedures that block the release or conversion of renin have major direct effects on peripheral blood pressure. Angiotensin may also act directly on the brain, although only a few target tissues that are not protected by the blood-brain barrier could be responsible for its actions.

The second hypothesis has been supported by numerous experimental findings. Angiotensin has been found to elicit drinking in sated animals when injected into three principal sites: 1) the preoptic region, 2) the AV3V, and 3) the subfornical organ.

The subfornical organ. The subfornical organ is a small organ that protrudes into the ventricular system near the junction of the lateral and the third ventricles. The neurons of this structure are on the blood side of the blood-brain barrier and are thus exposed to large peptides such as angiotensin. Many neurons in the subfornical organ are activated by intravenous injections or local iontophoretic applications of A-II, and this response is blocked by topical application of the competitive A-II blocker saralasin (Felix et al. 1986). The subfornical organ is widely believed to be the principal target of blood-borne A-II.

Injections into the subfornical organ of nanogram doses of A-II that are lower than those found effective intraventricularly have been reported to elicit drinking as well as vasopressin release and systemic pressor responses in the rat (J. B. Simpson et al. 1978) and many other species. Destruction of the subfornical organ or transection of its efferents reduces or completely abolishes the drinking and pressure responses to systemic A-II (Mangiapane and Simpson 1980; J. B. Simpson et al. 1978; Thrasher et al. 1982). Subfornical organ lesions also reduce the drinking response to polyethylene glycol-induced hypovolemia (J. B. Simpson et al. 1978) as well as systemic salt loads (Hosutt et al. 1981). Subfornical organ lesions have also been reported to reduce the drinking response to intraparenchymal as well as intracerebroventricular injections of A-II (Hoffman and Phillips 1976; J. B. Simpson and Routtenberg 1973), but this effect has been curiously variable. In view of these observations, it is surprising that subfornical organ lesions have little or no effect on deprivation-induced drinking (Simpson and Routtenberg 1973; Thrasher et al. 1982).

The AV3V, organum vasculosum of the lamina terminalis, and nucleus medianus. The second major site of thirst-related A-II action in the brain is comprised of the tissues surrounding the anterior aspects of the third ventricle. Several investigators have reported drinking as well as blood pressure effects after microinjections into the organum vasculosum of the lamina terminalis. The doses used in these experiments (as little as 50 fg in one experiment) are smaller by an order of magnitude than those effective in the subfornical organ (M. I. Phillips 1978; M. I. Phillips and Hoffman

1977). Lesions in the AV3V and organum vasculosum of the lamina terminalis and some or all of the nucleus medianus result in transient adipsia followed by a permanent inhibition of the drinking as well as pressure effects of systemic, intracerebroventricular, or intrapreoptic injections of A-II. These lesions also reduce drinking responses to systemic salt loads but have no effect on hypovolemic thirst (Buggy and Johnson 1977a, 1977b).

The preoptic area.   Historically, the first brain region found to be sensitive to angiotensin was the preoptic region that has been implicated in thirst and AVP release (Epstein et al. 1970). It was soon demonstrated that intracerebroventricular injections of even lower doses produced similar effects (Rolls et al. 1972), an observation that gave rise to the hypothesis that preoptic injections might elicit thirst because the hormone enters the ventricular system for transport to distant sites of action. Although experimental support for this interpretation was soon forthcoming (Johnson and Epstein 1975), some investigators have continued to discuss the involvement of a preoptic midbrain pathway in A-II drinking (Swanson et al. 1978). The principal empirical support for this conclusion is evidence that preoptic injections of A-II that do not gain access to ventricular spaces produce drinking (Richardson and Mogenson 1981; Swanson et al. 1978).

Angiotensin of peripheral origin does not enter cerebrospinal fluid or brain parenchyma (except at some circumventricular organisms). The proposed pathway thus would have to rely on endogenous angiotensin manufactured by neurons of the midbrain or preoptic region or both. This condition is plausible because renin-substrate, converting enzymes A-I and A-II, as well as angiotensinases that inactivate A-II, and specific angiotensin receptors have been found in the brain, notably in the hypothalamus and preoptic area. A-I and A-II binding sites have been specifically localized in nerve terminals in many of the brain structures implicated in thirst (M. I. Phillips 1987; Unger et al. 1986).

The concept of an endogenous angiotensin system finds support in numerous reports of drinking, in a variety of species, after intracranial injections of systemically ineffective doses of renin substrate, renin, or A-I (Epstein et al. 1970; Fitzsimons 1979; Fitzsimons et al. 1978).

The most widely accepted hypothesis about the action of angiotensin in the brain proposes a direct action of blood-borne angiotensin on neurons in the subfornical organ. This hypothesis is based primarily on the observation that many subfornical organ neurons respond to systemic A-II injections, the effect being blocked by topical application of the competitive angiotensin blocker saralasin (Felix et al. 1986; M. I. Phillips and Hoffman 1977). Saralasin injections into the subfornical organ also abolish the drinking response to systemic A-II (J. B. Simpson et al. 1978).

The nature of this interaction between A-II and neurons in the subfornical organ is not yet fully understood. Angiotensin is a powerful vasoconstrictor and could affect neurons in the highly vascular regions of the subfornical organ and, perhaps, AV3V (including the organum vasculosum of the lamina terminalis and nervi medianus) by acting on stretch receptors (Nicolaidis and Fitzsimons 1975). Although there is some evidence for this suggestion (see Fitzsimons 1979 for review), it is widely believed that the central action of A-II may best be understood by the assumption that it acts as a neurotransmitter or neuromodulator and thus affects neurons directly.

Neurons in the subfornical organ project to portions of the AV3V as well as the preoptic region, lateral hypothalamus, and paraventricular nucleus of the hypothalamus, which is the origin of the fibers of the median eminence that, in turn, gives rise to the portal connections to the anterior pituitary (Miselis 1981, Miselis et al. 1979). Reciprocal projections interconnect the hypothalamus and preoptic region with the AV3V and subfornical organ (Lind and Johnson 1982; Saper and Levisohn 1983).

It appears likely that the efferent projections of the subfornical organ may be angiotensinergic, which would account for the high sensitivity of the AV3V and preoptic region to local injections of angiotensin. There is, however, some evidence that the organum vasculosum of the lamina terminalis may itself be sensitive to angiotensin in the general circulation (Johnson and Buggy 1977) and may be responsible for the efficacy of intracerebroventricular angiotensin injections (Ganong 1984; M. I. Phillips 1987). The physiological significance of the proposed transport of A-II from cerebrospinal fluid into the AV3V is not readily apparent because circulating angiotensin does not, under normal circumstances, enter the ventricular system (Ganten et al. 1976).

Neuropharmacology of Thirst-Related Brain Mechanisms

Acetylcholine and carbachol. Microinjections of acetylcholine or the cholinomimetic carbachol (which produces more persistent activation of cholinergic receptors) elicit drinking (Grossman 1960) as well as decreased urine flow and increased urine concentration (N. E. Miller 1965). The renal effects are mediated by increased vasopressin release (Kühn 1974).

The effects of carbachol on drinking are behaviorally as well as pharmacologically specific. Carbachol elicits water-rewarded instrumental behaviors such as lever pressing. It also increases deprivation-induced water consumption, as well as the dipsogenic effects of systemic injections of hypertonic saline. Feeding in hungry rats is decreased (Grossman 1962a; N. E. Miller 1965).

The effects of carbachol are caused by its action on muscarinic receptor mechanisms (Stein and Seifter 1962). They are mimicked by injections of cholinesterase inhibitors that prolong the action of endogenous acetylcholine and are blocked by systemic or intracranial injections of acetylcholine receptor blockers such as atropine (Grossman 1962b; N. E. Miller 1965; Stein and Seifter 1962).

Intracranial atropine injections also reduce deprivation-induced drinking and the drinking response to systemic salt loads (Block and Fisher 1970; Grossman 1962b). Systemic injections of the cholinergic receptor blocker scopolamine reduces drinking to all cellular and extracellular thirst stimuli (Fisher 1973).

The central site of action of carbachol and related blocking agents has been the subject of controversy. Positive sites have been found throughout the upper brain stem as well as in the septum and the hippocampus (Fisher and Coury 1962). The resulting hypothesis of a diffuse representation of cholinergic thirst pathways is supported by the observation that atropine injections at sites along the proposed thirst circuit can block the drinking response to carbachol at other injection sites (Levitt and Fisher 1971). An alternative to this hypothesis is the notion that carbachol and atropine may diffuse into the ventricular system and act on the subfornical organ. This hypothesis is supported by the observations that injections of carbachol into the subfornical organ are effective at extremely low doses and lesions of the subfornical organ reduce the drinking response to carbachol injections elsewhere in the brain (J. B. Simpson and Routtenberg 1972). The fact that subfornical organ lesions do not block carbachol drinking completely indicates that the subfornical organ is not the only site of carbachol action and there is considerable evidence for effective carbachol injection sites in the medial preoptic area and AV3V (Swanson et al. 1978).

Carbachol-induced drinking is an exceptionally robust phenomenon in the rat. In other species, the effects are often weaker or absent, possibly resulting from such side effects as somnolence or extreme autonomic arousal that are incompatible with drinking (Hernandez-Peon et al. 1962; Myers 1964).

Catecholamines. Microinjections of α-adrenergic compounds such as norepinephrine into the hypothalamus and preoptic region inhibit deprivation-induced drinking, as well as drinking responses to systemic salt loads and intracranial carbachol (Leibowitz 1973; Setler 1975). The effects of norepinephrine on drinking are blocked by α-adrenergic blocking agents such as phentolamine but not by β-adrenergic blockers (Leibowitz 1980). Injections of norepinephrine into the lateral or third ventricle or into the supraoptic nucleus release vasopressin, the effect being blocked by α-adrenergic blocking agents (Kühn 1974; Urano and Kobayashi 1978).

Systemic injections of dopamine receptor blockers such as haloperidol reduce drinking in response to deprivation, hypertonic saline, polyethylene glycol, and isoproterenol (Fisher 1973). Concurrent injections of acetylcholine receptor blockers, such as scopolamine, inhibit extracellular thirst completely, whereas there is no additive effect with respect to deprivation- or salt-induced drinking (Fisher 1973). The site of action responsible for these effects is, as yet, unknown. Intracranial injections of dopamine receptor blockers inhibit A-II-induced drinking but have little or no effect on other thirst stimuli (Fisher 1973; Setler 1975).

Histamine.   Systemic injections of histamine elicit drinking in the rat (Leibowitz 1973) and reduce urine output, partly because of a direct action on the kidney and partly because of increased vasopressin release (Leibowitz 1979). The time course of histamine-induced drinking parallels a decrease in blood pressure and increased plasma renin activity (Leenen et al. 1975). However, this may not be the principal mechanism for the effect of histamine on drinking because nephrectomy reduces histamine-induced drinking only slightly (Gutman and Krausz 1973). Histamine injections into the supraoptic nucleus or periventricular nucleus also elicit drinking and antidiuresis. It is not clear whether the effects of systemic injection of histamine are caused by its action on these diencephalic mechanisms because the compound crosses the blood-brain barrier only in minute quantities. Systemic injections of a combination of H_1 and H_2 histamine receptor blockers (dexbrompheniramine and cimetidine, respectively) prevent the drinking response to systemic histamine and reduce periprandial drinking without affecting deprivation-induced drinking (Kraly 1986).

Amphibian peptides.   Several peptides have been extracted from amphibian skin that closely resemble peptides found in mammalian brains or intestines. Many of them have pronounced inhibitory effects on drinking when administered intracerebroventricularly in the rat.

One group of related substances, the tachikinins (eledoisin, physalaemin, and substance P) inhibit drinking responses to intracerebroventricular A-II or carbachol, as well as systemic salt loads and water deprivation. The tachikinin kassinin inhibits cellular thirst selectively. The tachikinins also release vasopressin. The effects of this group of peptides appear to be caused by their central action, because systemic injections are without effect. Intraparenchymal brain injections are most effective in the medial preoptic area, anterior hypothalamus, and subfornical organ. For a review of the extensive related literature see de Caro (1986) and de Caro and Micossi (1986).

A second group of antidipsogenic peptides consists of the bombesins (bombesin, ranatensin, and litorin). Intracerebro-

84 Water Balance in Schizophrenia

ventricular injections of extremely low doses of these peptides antagonize A-II-induced drinking. At much higher doses drinking responses to intracerebroventricular carbachol, salt loads, and water deprivation also are attenuated. In pigeons and ducks, the same peptides have pronounced dipsogenic effects.

Endogenous opioids and related compounds. Intracerebroventricular injections of the natural brain opioids leucine-enkephalin and methionine-enkephalin produce transient inhibitory effects on drinking, followed by persisting polydipsia accompanied by increased plasma renin activity that is a result of β-adrenergic stimulation of the kidney (de Caro 1986). A structurally related peptide, dermorphin, has a selective inhibitory effect on A-II drinking when administered at very low doses intracerebroventricularly. This effect appears to be caused by an action on the subfornical organ because even lower doses are effective when applied directly to the subfornical organ (Perfumi et al. 1986).

Morphine. Systemic injections of morphine also produce transient inhibitory effects on thirst followed by hyperdipsia that lasts several hours and is, in turn, followed by a prolonged period of reduced water intake. The effects of morphine are antagonized by the opioid receptor blocker naltrexone (Arslan et al. 1986).

Endogenous opioid receptor blockers such as naltrexone and naloxone reduce ad libitum water intake as well as drinking after deprivation, salt loads, polyethylene glycol-induced hypovolemia and angiotensin (Rowland 1982; Sanger 1983). These effects appear to be caused by a direct action of brain opiate receptors because intracranial injections of lower doses also produce hypodipsia (Czech et al. 1983).

Benzodiazepines. The minor tranquilizers of the diazepam family increase deprivation-induced drinking as well as drinking during cellular dehydration or extracellular hypovolemia. These effects are counteracted by benzodiazepine receptor blockers that do not affect deprivation-induced drinking and by opioid receptor blockers that do have an inhibitory effect on deprivation-induced thirst (Cooper 1986).

Prostaglandins. Prostaglandins are synthesized from essential fatty acids in all tissues, including the brain. They have numerous physiological functions of which many are not as yet fully understood. Prostaglandins can affect the regulation of fluid and sodium balances in several ways, including direct effects on renal glomeruli (J. B. Gross and Bartter 1973), systemic vasodilatation (Aiken and Vane 1973), and central pyretic effects (Fluharty 1981). We shall concentrate our attention on the interaction of prostaglandins of the E family with angiotensin-induced drinking.

Intracerebroventricular injections of prostaglandin E_1 or E_2 reduce the drinking response to systemic as well as central A-II. At much larger doses, drinking during polyethylene glycol-induced hypovolemia is also attenuated. The response to hypertonic saline, on the other hand, is spared (Kenney 1986). These intracerebroventricular injections also increase core temperature, and this effect appears to be correlated with the inhibition of drinking under some (Fluharty 1981) but not all (Kenney 1986) conditions.

These observations have led to the suggestion that the inhibition of A-II-induced drinking may be specifically related to an antagonistic interaction of the prostaglandins and A-II in the brain. The reduced response to hypovolemic drinking may reflect this interaction as well but may also be caused, at least in part, to the pyretic effects of the injections. According to this view, increases in plasma A-II act on extracellular thirst mechanisms in the subfornical organ (and possibly the AV3V as well) and thereby elicit drinking. Angiotensin also stimulates the synthesis and release of prostaglandin E, which reduces thirst either by a direct antagonistic action on angiotensin or by activating special satiety mechanisms in the brain.

Alternatively, the A-II-polyethylene glycol E interaction in the regulation of extracellular thirst might involve their respective vasomotor effects. Angiotensin produces systemic vasoconstriction, and it has been suggested that this might lead to the activation of subfornical organ neurons (Nicolaidis and Fitzsimons 1975). Prostaglandin E is a peripheral vasodilator in most species and has been shown to antagonize the vasoconstrictor action of A-II in the kidney (Aiken and Vane 1973). It may do so in the subfornical organ and thus attenuate extracellular thirst.

Attempts to test the general hypothesis that an antagonistic A-II-polyethylene glycol E interaction is responsible for the termination of extracellular thirst have produced inconsistent results. Systemic or intracerebroventricular injections of prostaglandin synthesis inhibitors have been reported to increase, decrease, or have no effect on the magnitude of A-II drinking. For a review of this literature see Kenney (1986).

Systemic injections of prostaglandin E_1 or E_2 inhibit A-II drinking much as do intracerebroventricular injections. However, they also attenuate drinking elicited by cellular dehydration, even at low doses of polyethylene glycol E, and have only small effects, at very high doses, on drinking elicited by polyethylene glycol. In contrast to the pyretic effects of intracerebroventricular prostaglandins, systemic injections reduce body temperature (Kenney et al. 1981). It should be noted that systemically administered polyethylene glycol E does not enter into the brain, although an action on the subfornical organ or other circumventricular structures may, of course, result in an indirect action on the brain.

CONCLUSIONS

Thirst is a general sensation that arises as a consequence of obligatory water loss from the body. However, we drink more fluid than necessary to replenish body fluids, to wet the mouth during meals, to cool off when it is hot, and to enjoy desirable taste sensations.

We thus regulate body fluids mainly by urine excretion. After a period of deprivation, humans drink just enough to meet physiological need and stop in response to oral and gastric satiety cues before the body's fluid balance has been reestablished. Although oral and gastric satiety signals play an important role under normal circumstances, they are not essential to normal body fluid regulation.

Body fluids are contained in two compartments, intracellular water and extracellular (interstitial fluid and blood plasma). The two compartments are separated by a semipermiable cell membrane that permits movement of water and some solutes but excludes salts such as sodium from cells. When water or solutes are lost from the cellular or extracellular fluid compartment, water moves into the compartment containing the higher concentration by a process of osmosis.

Water and salt are continually lost from extracellular stores because of evaporation, digestion, and urine formation. This loss results in hypovolemia that can be a primary thirst stimulus when large quantities of fluids are lost to diarrhea, bleeding, or prolonged water deprivation. Because proportionately more water than solutes is lost, the concentration of solutes in extracellular fluid increases during water deprivation. The resulting osmotic forces move water out of cells, thus partially restoring the extracellular fluid volume while producing cellular dehydration.

When water is ingested after deprivation, extracellular fluid is diluted, thus reversing the osmotic pressure relations between the extracellular and cellular fluid compartment. This effect causes water to move into cells and thus eliminates cellular dehydration thirst. Hypovolemia is not completely reversed by the ingestion of water. Complete restoration of the body's fluid balance requires the ingestion of sodium salt that permits the retention of fluid in the extracellular compartment.

Cellular hydration is monitored by osmoreceptors in the preoptic region of the brain. Information about the volume of extracellular fluid reaches the brain by two means. Hypovolemia increases the concentration of angiotensin in the circulation and stimulates the vascular stretch receptors. Angiotensin releases aldosterone from the adrenal gland and acts on the cells of the subfornical region of the brain. Other cells in the diencephalon respond to neural signals from the vascular receptors. Both signals stimulate thirst as well as vasopressin release.

The brain mechanisms that control thirst are concentrated in the tissues surrounding the anterior third ventricle. Different aspects of thirst are controlled by several structures in that region. Some (the lateral preoptic area and the supraoptic and paraventricular nuclei) contain osmoreceptors that mediate behavioral and renal responses to cellular dehydration. Others, such as the subfornical organ and the AV3V, serve as receptor sites for angiotensin and mediate drinking as well as the renal responses to extracellular hypovolemia. Still others, such as the zona incerta and the lateral hypothalamus, serve more general integrative functions related to drinking.

Chapter 4

Cellular Regulation of Water Transport: Role of Plasma Membrane Structure and Function

Sahebarao P. Mahadik, Ph.D., Sukdeb Mukherjee, M.D.,* and Hemant S. Kelkar, Ph.D.

Total body water is maintained within the physiological range by a balance of intake and excretion. Cell plasma membrane regulates the distribution of 80% of the total body water between two compartments: 60% in intracellular and 20% in interstitial (extracellular) fluids. The remaining 20% of water is distributed between bone (5%), connective tissue (7.5%), and plasma (7.5%), and this remains fairly constant even under altered physiological circumstances (I. S. Edelman and Leibman 1959; Woodbury 1974). The distribution of body water between intracellular and extracellular fluids is determined by two forces: hydrostatic pressure and osmotic pressure (A. C. Brown 1974). The regulation of intracellular water is a function of the cell membrane of each individual cell (Leaf 1970), but the water content of the extracellular fluid is determined by plasma water, which ultimately is regulated by the kidney (M.B. Goldman 1991).

In the body, hydrostatic pressure in the vascular bed influences the water distribution between plasma and extracellular fluids but does not have any influence on water distribution across the cell plasma membrane because it is counterbalanced within the

---

*Deceased

89

vascular system. Therefore, only the osmotic force determines the water distribution across cell plasma membrane. Because water can diffuse freely across all cell plasma membranes, the extracellular and intracellular fluids remain in osmotic equilibrium and, hence, the water potential remains the same (Maffly and Leaf 1959). As a result, the distribution of the body water between the intracellular fluid and the extracellular fluid is determined by osmotically active components in each compartment. Sodium ions (142 mEq/L) are the extracellular osmotically active ions, and the potassium ions (140 mEq/L) are the intracellular osmotically active ions. Although the cell membrane is permeable to these ions, their movement across the plasma membrane is regulated by the Na^+-K^+ pump (Sweadner and Goldin 1980), which is present in high concentrations in plasma membranes of each cell type in the body (Avruch and Wallach 1971). The activity of this pump is dependent on the plasma membrane structure (biochemical and biophysical), which is determined by the composition and distribution of proteins and lipids, as well as by membrane interaction of several peptide hormones. In neural membranes, the Na^+-K^+ pump is regulated also by some neurotransmitter receptor-mediated processes. Alterations in these membrane-mediated processes can contribute to altered osmotic balance and thereby result in altered cellular water transport and associated pathophysiology. These processes also are affected by the intake of water and salt by oral ingestion and their excretion by the kidney.

The physiological regulation and mechanisms of water intake and excretion are complex and will be discussed briefly to explain the role of cell membrane in water transport. It is possible to study some of these processes in vitro in isolated cell membrane preparations. To understand the cellular water transport, it is helpful to understand cell membrane structure and its relationship to function. We describe the general procedures for isolating cell plasma membranes and studying their biochemical and biophysical properties. Plasma membrane structure plays an important role in its functions, particularly ionic transport, which regulates the water distribution across plasma membrane, and underlying regulatory mechanisms. These processes will be discussed in reference to plasma membranes of tubular cells of kidney and neuronal cells in the brain, because dysfunction of either of these organs can lead to disordered water balance in a variety of clinical conditions, including psychiatric disorders. This altered water balance may eventually lead to multiple disorders, such as polydipsia and polyuria with or without hyponatremia (Berl and Schrier 1986; Sterns and Spital 1990), which often are observed in psychiatric conditions, particularly in schizophrenia (Barlow and De Wardener 1959; Ferrier 1985; M.B. Goldman 1991; Illowsky and Kirch 1988; Kirch et al. 1985; Lapierre et al. 1990; Singh et al. 1985; Sleeper and Jellinek 1936; Vieweg et al. 1985a). This acute water imbalance can produce a multisystem failure that can result in convulsions, coma, and death (Blum and Friedland 1983; Blum et al. 1983; Jose et al. 1979; Kushnir et al. 1990; Resnick and Patterson 1969; Rowntree 1923; Vieweg et al. 1985a). We also briefly discuss the research strategies for investigating underlying mechanisms and possible treatment strategies.

BIOCHEMICAL AND BIOPHYSICAL PROPERTIES OF CELL PLASMA MEMBRANE

The most satisfactory model for plasma membrane structure, the fluid mosaic model, was provided by Singer and Nicolson (1972). This model postulated that the phospholipids are arranged in a bilayer to form a fluid microenvironment where individual phospholipids can move freely, thus endowing the bilayer with fluidity, flexibility, and characteristically high electrical resistance and relative impermeability to charged molecules. This model further postulated that membrane proteins are partially or fully embedded in this bilayer and can move laterally in two dimensions. The biochemical composition (proteins and lipids) of cell membrane determines its biophysical properties (fluidity and integrity), and together they regulate (determine) membrane functions, particularly ion transport, which influences water transport across the plasma membrane. The schematic diagram of the cell plasma membrane structure that includes lipid bilayer with proteins embedded in it is shown in Figure 4–1.

Outside (Interstitial space)

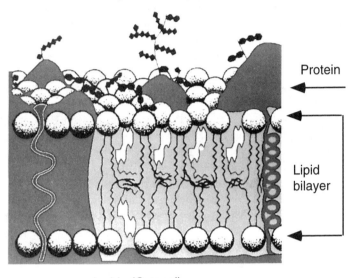

Inside (Cytosol)

Figure 4–1. Schematic diagram of cell plasma membrane structure. Diagram shows a lipid bilayer with lipid head groups (circles) of outer layer located at the outer surface and that of the inner layer located at the inner surface in contact with cytosol. Fatty acids (zig-zag lines) bound to lipids make the core. Membrane proteins (receptors, ion channels, ion transporters, enzymes, and regulatory proteins) in different sizes, shapes, and orientations embedded in lipid bilayer are shown as large dark masses. Some proteins and lipids with attached polysaccharides (shown as chains of filled hexagons, hexoses) on the outer surface, called glycoproteins and glycolipids, respectively, are also shown embedded in lipid bilayer.

Isolation of Plasma Membranes

Advances in methodologies for isolating cell plasma membranes from various tissues have aided the investigation of the structural basis of cell-specific membrane functions and investigation of the underlying regulatory processes. A large number of published procedures for isolation of cell plasma membranes from different tissues have been reported that differ slightly as a result of varying degree of connective tissue (Findley and Evans 1990). All procedures involve two main steps: disruption of tissue and the cells and separation of various subcellular organelles and their membranes from cell plasma membranes. Isolation of cell membranes from the kidney is somewhat elaborate, because membranes along the microvilli are not homogeneous (Aronson 1978; Booth and Kenny 1974; Kinne and Schwartz 1978). Isolation of neural membranes is simpler, but the plasma membrane fraction is heterogeneous because it represents membranes from different neuronal and glial populations (Mahadik et al. 1978; Tamir et al. 1976; Whittaker 1966). Typically, plasma membranes are separated by differential and density gradient centrifugation followed by, if necessary, aqueous two-phase partitioning or preparative free-flow electrophoresis (see Findley and Evans 1990 for references). Because the plasma membrane of each cell type in the body is unique, the homogeneity of isolated fraction can be assessed using cell-specific markers as well as general biochemical and biophysical plasma membrane markers.

Biochemical Properties

The unique chemical composition of the cell membrane of each cell type in the body allows the cells to carry out specialized functions as well as some common functions, such as ion transport. Plasma membranes from different cell types contain a wide range of proteins and lipids (e.g., kidney membranes contain 60% protein and 40% lipids, and myelin membranes contain 20% protein and 80% lipids) (Findley and Evans 1990; Finean et al. 1966; van Deenen 1966). Plasma membranes with a higher lipid-to-protein ratio, such as neural membranes, exhibit higher electrical resistance than membranes with a lower ratio, such as those from the liver and kidney. Therefore, neural plasma membranes can better control ionic transport across the membrane, which allows rapid generation of the action potential and its propagation over long distances without a significant decrease in amplitude. Also, this characteristic property helps to maintain the stable osmotic balance between extracellular and intracellular compartments and thereby protects the cell from excess intracellular water accumulation and cell swelling. Membrane proteins constitute ion channels, receptors, and regulatory proteins. The surface membrane proteins (receptors) interact with the microenvironment (transmitters, hormones, toxins, and so forth) and can further influence the membrane functions and thereby affect the water transport (see below). Changes in plasma membrane proteins can be analyzed either by determining their functional activity, such as enzymatic activity or ion transport, or by computer-assisted quantitative densitometric analysis of the patterns after separation using two-dimensional slab gel electrophoresis (Garrels 1983). Isolated plasma membrane fractions provide a source of membrane proteins that can be studied in vitro for their structural as well as functional properties, for example, transport of Na^+ and K^+ by Na^+-K^+ pump in isolated renal microvillus membranes (Katz 1982) or neurotransmitter functions, such as dopamine receptor mechanisms in synaptic plasma membranes (Glowinski et al. 1988).

The role of membrane lipids in membrane function is complex. The content and distribution of phospholipids maintain membrane integrity and fluidity necessary for the optimum function of membrane ionic pumps and receptors and also directly regulate their activities. Particularly, the type and content of lipid-bound fatty acids, and the ratio of saturated to unsaturated fatty acids, play important roles in determining fluidity as well as regulating membrane functional proteins. Also, receptor-mediated increase in the metabolism of these lipids leads to functionally active second messengers (e.g., arachidonic acid, prostaglandins, and leukotrienes) that can further influence cellular physiological processes, including ion transport mechanisms. The membrane glycolipids are generally localized asymmetrically and extend an attached carbohydrate moiety on the membrane surface, which can act as receptors for hormones and toxins and can further influence the membrane ion transport. The alterations in plasma membrane lipids and associated fatty acids are studied by their separation on thin-layer chromatography followed by analysis of fatty acid using gas chromatography. Any alterations in this delicate balance between lipids and protein in plasma membrane can cause membrane dysfunction and lead to pathophysiological consequences.

Biophysical Properties

Because the chemical composition of the cell membrane determines its biophysical structure, the plasma membrane of each cell must have unique biophysical properties. These properties are studied by measurement of membrane fluidity by fluorescence polarization and structural integrity and phase transition using membrane enzyme activities as a function of temperature (Lakowicz 1983). Membrane fluidity and structural integrity regulate the functional activities of membrane proteins and lipids. Conversely, changes in these parameters are a reflection of the alterations in chemical composition of the membrane. Although alterations in biophysical parameters are not sensitive and cell specific, they provide an approximation of membrane change with relatively fast and simple procedures, whereas biochemical analyses involve lengthy and elaborate procedures.

PLASMA MEMBRANE FUNCTIONS IN CELLULAR WATER TRANSPORT

Ion Transport

The most relevant function of cell plasma membrane in regulation of cellular water transport is the maintenance of ionic balance, particularly that of Na^+ and K^+ between extracellular fluid and the intracellular fluid compartments. This function is possible because of the concentration differences of Na^+ and K^+ and the electric potential difference between intracellular and extracellular fluids, which are results of slow diffusion of minute fractions of these ions through water- and energy-dependent transport (active transport) (Woodbury 1974). The transport of Na^+ and K^+ by plasma membrane is predominantly an active transport by Na^+-K^+ pump. In renal microvillus membrane, the uptake of Na^+ also is affected by a Na^+-H^+ exchanger (Green and Giebisch 1975; Kinsella and Aronson 1980; Murer et al. 1976). In addition, there is some diffusion and exchange of Na^+ and Ca^{++}, but their contribution to influence the cellular water transport is minimal (A. C. Brown 1974). These processes are common to most cells of the body. However, in tissues such as brain, different cells may have different rates of ion transport to accommodate their differential activity needs. This difference may require a fine adjustment of active ion transport by the cell membrane to meet the needs of the particular type of cell. The mechanisms involved in these processes are discussed later. These processes are further influenced by interaction of environmental factors with their membrane receptors that can result in changes in the receptor-mediated regulatory processes.

Response to Microenvironment

Response to microenvironment is one of the most important functions of the cell plasma membrane because interactions between extracellular microenvironmental factors and cell membrane surface receptors contribute to cellular adoption to physiological demands. Cell membrane ion transport can be either blocked or enhanced by the interaction with extracellular environmental factors (hormones, neurotransmitters, and toxins) that can affect water transport. In the kidney, several antidiuretic hormones (arginine vasopressin, aldosterone, renin-angiotensin) can bind to membrane receptors and affect salt and water excretion (Masiak and Naylor 1985). Other hormones can also influence kidney cell membrane reabsorption or secretion (Katz 1982; M.B. Goldman 1991). In the brain, action of neurotransmitters at receptors can influence membrane ionic transport and affect cellular water transport. For example, increased concentration of the excitatory amino acid glutamate can lead to increased intracellular Na^+ and Ca^{++} and thereby cell swelling and even death (Choi 1987). Similarly, enterotoxins by their action on membrane surface receptors in intestinal brush border cells may cause the loss of cellular water by depleting cellular levels of Na^+. This reduction clearly indicates that cellular water transport can be greatly influenced by alterations of membrane ion transport function owing to interactions between extracellular environmental factors and plasma membrane surface receptors.

Receptor-Mediated Transfer of Information

Plasma membrane structure and function also are influenced by processes associated with receptor-mediated (hormone or neurotransmitter) transfer of information. These processes include activation of lipases or cyclases, protein kinases, phosphodiesterases, and generation of second messengers (adenosine 3',5'-monophosphate [cAMP], cyclic guanosine monophosphate, Ca^{++}, inositol triphosphate, and arachidonic acid). In neuronal membranes, these processes trigger a cascade of Na^+ and K^+ transport mechanisms (i.e., activation of ion transporters and ion gated channels). Most of these receptor-mediated processes involve the guanidine nucleotide regulatory protein. Binding of guanosine triphosphate to this protein leads to dissociation of the hormone from its receptor and activation of adenyl cyclase (Kurokawa 1989). The two receptor systems are important in water regulation: osmoreceptors in the hypothalamus and the arginine vasopressin (AVP) receptors in the kidney.

The osmoreceptors are located in the hypothalamus near the cell bodies of the neurohypophysis. These cells respond to 1%–2% change in plasma osmolality (normal plasma osmolality is 287 mOsm/kg water x 2%) by influencing thirst and AVP release. The AVP levels drop below detectable levels when plasma osmolality falls below 280 mOsm/kg. It has been suggested that pathological alterations in the functional properties of these osmoreceptors can result in a variety of well-characterized disorders of salt and water balance (Robertson et al. 1976). However, the biochemical processes that determine the functions of the osmoreceptors are unclear.

In the kidney, AVP binds to V_2 receptors that are localized in the basolateral plasma membranes and coupled to adenylate cyclase. In isolated nephron segments, AVP-sensitive adenylate cyclase is found both in the thick ascending limb of Henley's loop and in the collecting tubules. It has been shown that several physiological substances, such as prostaglandin E_2, α-adrenergic catecholamines, and somatostatin, act on the activation of AVP-dependent cyclase and modulate the action of AVP on permeability of the collecting tubules. Prostaglandin E_2, which is produced by medullary interstitial cells and collecting tubules, has been shown to inhibit the AVP-dependent increase in water permeability in collecting tubules, possibly by suppressing cAMP formation. It also can impair the generation and maintenance of medullary hypertonicity. It is interesting that AVP seems to stimulate prostaglandin E_2 production, probably via V_1 receptors in renal interstitial cells and collecting tubules. This AVP action can be regarded as a local feedback system regulating AVP action on the collecting tubules (Kurokawa 1989).

Under physiological conditions cell plasma membrane ionic regulatory processes are tightly regulated so that altered ionic changes are rapidly reversed and do not affect the water distribution between intracellular and extracellular fluid compartments. Under pathophysiological conditions, when these receptor-mediated processes are overstimulated, for example, during ischemia in the brain, they lead to cellular ionic imbalance, which, in turn, can result in altered cellular water transport (Katzman et al. 1977).

PLASMA MEMBRANE MECHANISMS FOR REGULATION OF CELLULAR WATER TRANSPORT

Na⁺-K⁺ Pumps

A major Na^+-K^+ pump is the enzyme, Na^+-K^+-dependent Mg^{++}-activated adenosine triphosphate phosphohydrolase (Na^+-K^+-ATPase) (Jorgensen 1980; Schuurmans-Stekhoven and Bonting 1981). It is present in plasma membranes of all cell types in vertebrates (Avruch and Wallach 1971; Skou 1957), and its primary role is to pump two Na^+ out and one K^+ in for each ATP molecule hydrolyzed (Sweadner 1979; Sweadner and Goldin 1980; Whittam and Wheeler 1970) as well as membrane transport activity-dependent energy utilization in plasma membranes (Mata et al. 1980). By keeping intracellular Na^+ low, the cells are protected from excess intracellular water accumulation and cell swelling. Na^+-K^+-ATPase activity is dependent on its membrane lipid microenvironment (Kimelberg 1977; Tanaka and Teruya 1973). Because the lipid concentration and distribution determine membrane integrity and fluidity, change in the level of Na^+-K^+-ATPase activity is a good indicator of plasma membrane dysfunction (Grishman and Barnett 1973; W. E. Harris and Stahl 1985; Kimelberg 1977; Mahadik et al. 1992).

In the kidney, Na^+-K^+-ATPase is found in large amounts and is responsible for 50% of Na^+ and K^+ transport (Katz 1982). It is localized on the basolateral aspect of the renal tubular cell where its localization is predicated by the direction of the electrochemical potential. Methodological advances in the isolation of homogeneous tubular segments of the nephron (Burg et al. 1966) and the ultramicromethod of enzymatic analysis (Lowry and Passoneau 1972) have made it possible to understand the relationship between Na^+_K^+-ATPase activity and Na^+ transport in the single tubule. It has been shown that this enzyme participates in chronic adaptation of the kidney to altered Na^+ absorption and K^+ secretory load (Silva et al. 1977), and it can also promote "secondary" active transport processes that use the electropotential across plasma membrane or the sodium gradient generated by the Na^+-K^+ pump (Sachs 1977). Furthermore, Na^+-K^+-ATPase activity in the kidney is regulated by several hormones: mineralo- and glucocorticoids, thyroid, insulin, catecholamines, and others (for details see Katz 1982). Finally, the roles of vanadium and "natriuretic hormone(s)" in the inhibition of this enzyme suggest that these factors also may play a role in certain pathological situations (Bello-Reuss et al. 1979; Gonick et al. 1977).

There are three isozymes, each one with a distinct catalytic α-subunit (α-1, α-2, and α-3) of Na^+-K^+-ATPase (Fambrough 1988; Filuk et al. 1989; Herrera et al. 1987; Hsu and Guidotti 1989; Schneider et al. 1988; Shull et al. 1986; Sweadner 1989). Each is a separate enzyme with large differences in their kinetic characteristics. The kidney Na^+-K^+-ATPase exists as only α-1 isozyme, which was previously described as α, with low affinity to ouabain and high Km for Na^+ and low Km for K^+ (Sweadner and Goldin 1980). In the brain, all three isozymes have been identified using messenger RNA blot hybridization (Filuk et al. 1989; Schneider et al. 1988) and monoclonal antibodies (Urayama et al. 1989). α-1 is similar to enzyme in the kidney; α-2 and α-3 are catalytically similar to the previously described α^+ (high affinity to ouabain) (Sweadner 1979; Urayama and Sweadner 1988). α-3 is primarily associated with neurons (Schneider et al. 1988) and has a cellular distribution similar to α-2 (Filuk et al. 1989; Urayama et al. 1989); α-2 and α-3 constitute more than 65% of the total Na^+-K^+-ATPase in adult rat brain (Hieber et al. 1991; Uramaya and Sweadner 1988). This differential cellular distribution of kinetically distinct isozymes of Na^+-K^+-ATPase with their differential affinity to hormones and neurotransmitters is considered to meet specific physiological need to maintain the ionic homeostasis.

Changes in Na^+-K^+-ATPase activity have been implicated in the pathogenesis of hypertension, obesity, affective disorders, and certain manifestations of the uremic syndrome (Katz 1982). Similar studies on activity levels of Na^+-K^+-ATPase and other ion pumps (Besarab et al. 1976; Sachs 1977) in plasma membranes of kidney, erythrocyte, and brain tissues from psychotic patients with disorders of water transport have provided information on the role of membrane Na^+ and K^+ transport and its effect on cellular water transport.

Role of Plasma Sodium

Sodium in plasma is the main ion contributing to plasma osmolality. The osmolality of Na^+ salts can be calculated by multiplying plasma [Na^+] by 1.88 (I. S. Edelman et al. 1958). Because the plasma [Na^+] is 137–145 mEq/L and the [glucose] is 60–100 mg/dL, fasting, the effective plasma osmolality is 270–285 mOsm/kg. The effective plasma (and extracellular fluid) osmolality is the osmoles acting to hold water within the extracellular space. Urea is an ineffective osmole. This is expressed by the equations (I. S. Edelman et al. 1958)

$$\text{Effective } P_{osm} = 2 \times \text{plasma } [Na^+] + [glucose] \div 18;$$

$$\text{Plasma } [Na^+] \, \alpha \, \frac{[Na^+] + [K^+]}{\text{Total body water}}$$

In a clinical situation involving polydipsia, hyponatremia will occur only if retention of ingested water occurs, and the converse will be true for hypernatremia. This effect suggests that in psychotic patients, hyponatremia (serum osmolality is 266–277 mOsm/kg versus 285–295 mOsm/kg in nonpsychotic persons) may result from reduced water excretion by the kidney along with increased water intake (polydipsia).

Sustained hyponatremia may eventually decrease [Na⁺] in the extracellular fluid, which will result in decrease in the osmolality of extracellular fluid. This decrease can cause cellular water transport into the cell, particularly brain cells, which produce symptoms associated with hypoosmolality of extracellular fluid.

Role of Plasma Antidiuretic Hormones

As discussed earlier, the levels of plasma antidiuretic hormones are regulated by plasma osmolality. An increase in plasma tonicity will stimulate thirst and the osmoreceptors on the posterior pituitary cells releasing arginine vasopressin, and reduced plasma osmolality will suppress thirst and lower the secretion of vasopressin (M.B. Goldman 1991; Robertson et al. 1976; Verney 1947).

In the kidney, several antidiuretic hormones (arginine vasopressin, aldosterone, renin-angiotensin) can bind to membrane receptors and affect salt and water excretion (Masiak and Naylor 1985). The action of vasopressin on microvillus tubular cell membrane receptors that are either linked (Morel 1981) or not linked to adenyl cyclase (Doucet and Katz 1981) can lead to increased sodium and water reabsorption. Other hormones (supra) can also influence the kidney cell membrane reabsorption or secretion (Daniel and Heinrich 1990; Goldman 1991; Katz 1982; Kurokawa 1989). All of these processes are regulated by plasma membrane surface receptors.

MECHANISMS OF WATER IMBALANCE AND CELL PLASMA MEMBRANE

Psychiatric Patients

A brief summary is provided below to address the possible involvement of cell plasma membrane abnormalities in water imbalance. The etiology and pathophysiology of polydipsia and hyponatremia, and subsequent water intoxication in psychotic patients, is complex (M.B. Goldman 1991). There appear to be at least two stages involved: 1) polydipsia and associated hyponatremia and 2) complications of hyponatremia. Each of these stages may have a discrete pathophysiological basis. Polydipsia seems to be the first disturbance, leading subsequently to hyponatremia and eventually water intoxication (Blum et al. 1983; Jose and Perez-Cruet 1979; Vieweg et al. 1984a, 1986c). Several mechanisms have been proposed. In a controlled study, Goldman and coworkers concluded that psychiatric patients with polydipsia and hyponatremia have unexplained defects in the secretion of vasopressin, osmoregulation of water intake, and urinary dilution (M. B. Goldman et al. 1988). The syndrome of inappropriate antidiuretic hormone secretion has been suggested as a major etiological factor (Bartter and Schwartz 1967).

Plasma vasopressin levels are reported to be high in psychotic patients (Emsley et al. 1989; M.B. Goldman 1991; Raskind et al. 1975, 1978), which suggests that either there is a defect in regulation of osmoreceptors by plasma osmolality (reduced osmotic threshold for vasopressin secretion) or a defect in the suppression of thirst, or both. There is also some evidence that the sensitivity of the kidney to vasopressin may be increased, thereby increasing water reabsorption (Goldman 1991; M. B. Goldman et al. 1988; Robertson et al. 1976). In polydipsic patients, when the capacity of the kidney to excrete water is exceeded by excessive water intake, water retention and subsequent hyponatremia can develop.

This raises a question: Is water intoxication the result of chronic and sustained polydipsia and hyponatremia? Sustained polydipsia as well as hyponatremia may lead to water intoxication and associated complications, which include increased body weight, polyuria, psychosis, seizure, coma, congestive heart failure, osteopenia, and even death (Blum and Friedland 1983; Blum et al. 1983; Delva and Crammer 1988; Delva et al. 1989). As discussed earlier, prolonged hyponatremia can cause reduced extracellular osmolality, which will cause water transport into the cell. Although initially the cell membrane will be able to regulate the osmolality of intracellular fluid relative to extracellular osmolality, over long periods of time that capacity may impair and result in cell swelling. It has been shown that neurons exposed to hypoosmotic conditions in culture swell and accumulate intracellular calcium (Sanchez-Olea et al. 1993), which can lead to a cell death (Siesjo and Bengtsson 1989). The increase in intracellular water (cell swelling), particularly in the brain, can result in headache, ataxia, tremor, nausea, vomiting, confusion, lethargy, coma, convulsions, and death (Jose and Perez-Cruet 1979; Kushnir et al. 1990; Resnick and Patterson 1969; Vieweg et al. 1985a). These clinical symptoms are similar to those seen after hypoxic central nervous system stroke, which results in brain edema (Katzman et al. 1977). Central nervous system disorders are the most prominent clinical manifestations of disorders of fluid, electrolyte, and acid-base metabolism (Arieff and Schmidt 1980). In other tissues, increased intracellular water can impair cell functions and lead to organ dysfunction. This evidence suggests that, when sustained, water intoxication can lead to widespread cellular dysfunction, including cellular death in both neural and nonneural tissues.

Schizophrenia

Although there is no direct evidence that cell plasma membrane abnormalities are involved in the altered osmotic response of the neurohypophysis, the enhanced response of kidney to antidiuretic hormone and the eventual failure of kidney function during acute stages of water intoxication (polydipsia/polyurea and acute hyponatremia) suggest that this possibility is worth considering. The role of the cell plasma membrane in polydipsia and hyponatremia has been suggested from studies in Rhesus monkeys. It was reported that offspring of mothers fed until term with diets deficient in ω-3 fatty acids, critical components of both neural and nonneural cell plasma membrane phospholipids, showed increased water intake and output of urine (Reisbick et al. 1990). Later these investigators reported that the monkeys had increased fluid intake despite normal drinking frequency and preferences, normal urine analysis and clinical serum values, ability to concentrate urine, and absence of skin and renal pathology (Reisbick et al. 1991). In another study the investigators found that postnatal deficiency by itself was sufficient for the effects (Reisbick et al. 1992).

Also, the levels of ω-3 fatty acid in red blood cells were significantly lower in this study, suggesting generalized membrane abnormalities. In addition to polydipsia in monkeys, ω-3 fatty acid
deficiency has been found to cause visual impairment and abnormal electroretinograms (Neuringer et al. 1986).

The low levels of ω-3 fatty acids have been found to alter the
membrane structure and function (Brenner 1984) and the metabolism of prostaglandins and other eicosanoids (Granstrom 1987;
Sprecher 1986). Altered membrane structure can affect the cell
membrane surface, which plays a critical role through its interaction with the extracellular microenvironment in neurodevelopment
(G. M. Edelman 1976). There is compelling evidence that fatty acids play a critical role in brain and behavioral development (Wainwright 1992). In particular, the long-chain polyunsaturated ω-3 fatty
acid docosahexaenoic acid is critical in early brain developmental
and maturational events, especially around the time of birth (Wainwright 1992). The evidence suggests that polydipsia in schizophrenic patients may be a late result of preexisting generalized
membrane abnormalities that adversely affected neurodevelopment and lowered the threshold for later complications.

Evidence is increasing to support the view that neurodevelopmental complications contribute to the pathophysiology of schizophrenia (Feinberg 1982; Fish et al. 1992; Mukherjee et al. 1991;
Roberts 1989; Weinberger 1987). The increased prevalence of
neurointegrative disorders in infants at risk for psychiatric disorders and some of the neuropathological findings in the central nervous system support the notion of generalized developmental
complications in schizophrenia (reviewed by Fish et al. 1992). Generalized cell membrane abnormalities can explain such widespread
subtle developmental dysfunctions.

There is increasing evidence for generalized plasma membrane
abnormalities in schizophrenia (Crayton and Meltzer 1979;
Hitzemann et al. 1984; Mahadik et al. 1991; Rotrosen and Wolkin
1987; Stevens 1972), including tyrosine transport both in skin fibroblasts (Hagenfeldt et al. 1987) and across the blood-brain barrier
(Wiesel 1991). Altered phospholipids and associated fatty acids have
been found in red blood cells (Horrobin et al. 1992) as well as in
postmortem frontal cortex tissue from schizophrenic patients
(Horrobin et al. 1991). It has also been suggested that the alterations

in cell membrane lipids are reflected in changes in fatty acids in plasma phospholipids in schizophrenic patients from a crossnational population (Horrobin et al. 1989; Kaiya et al. 1991) and in twins (Bates et al. 1992). A role of essential fatty acids and abnormal levels of metabolites of released fatty acids (eicosanoids and prostaglandins) also has been suggested in schizophrenia (Feldberg 1976; Horrobin 1990, 1992; Van Kammen et al. 1989).

General plasma membrane pathology discussed earlier can contribute to altered processing of sensory information, typical of psychoses, by altering neuronal networks during development as well as by affecting the magnitude and the efficiency of conductance of membrane potential. Membrane potential is dependent on its structure and function. Also, the membrane pathology hypothesis can accommodate the dysfunction of multiple neurotransmitters, including dopamine receptor-mediated transfer of information, through a cascade of biochemical events. Altered membrane structure (lipids and proteins), and consequently fluidity, can change transmitter affinity to its receptor as well as the number of receptors, second messenger systems that involve G proteins, activation of lipases and release of fatty acids, activation of adenyl and guanyl cyclases and formation of cyclic nucleotides, activation of protein kinases, and phosphorylation of membrane proteins. Alterations in these processes can result in altered transport of ions across the plasma membrane (Na^+, K^+, Ca^{++}) and can affect the membrane potential, transmitter release, and expression of immediate early genes. The released fatty acids can be metabolized generating prostaglandins, thromboxanes, and leukotrienes, which can further influence the neuronal activities (Horrobin 1990; Van Kammen et al. 1989). Prostaglandins also play an important role in renal blood flow, renin secretion, sodium secretion, and water secretion (Daniel and Heinrich 1990). Some of these membrane processes may be associated with altered osmoreceptor response in posterior pituitary and the AVP receptor-mediated regulation of kidney function.

Research Strategies

As discussed above, disorders of water balance are common in schizophrenic patients, but not every patient has them. However, plasma membrane abnormalities seem to exist in both neural and nonneural cells in most of these patients. Also, the monkey model of polydipsia indicates that developmental deficiency of ω-3 fatty acids, early in life, can lead to polydipsia. These observations raise a number of questions: 1) Is there a specific membrane abnormality that contributes to water imbalance in schizophrenia, or is it a result of generalized membrane dysfunction? 2) If membrane abnormality is preexisting, why does polydipsia develop much later, many years after the onset of schizophrenia? 3) Do the generalized membrane abnormalities contribute to complications of water intoxication?

To answer these questions, a series of experiments can be done on the regulation of water transport in schizophrenic patients with and without disorders of water imbalance using various cell models such as red blood cells, lymphocytes, and skin fibroblasts. Red blood cells and lymphocytes have been used to study ionic transport and neurotransmitter receptor membrane mechanisms (Stahl 1985); however, their use is limited because they are highly differentiated and committed to specialized functions. Skin fibroblasts in culture are relatively undifferentiated and are well suited to study dynamic regulatory processes in response to the microenvironment because they express several ionic pumps and hormonal and neurotransmitter receptors that are present on both neural and nonneural cell membranes (Edelstein and Breakefield 1980; Giller 1980). It is possible that in the subgroup of schizophrenic patients who develop disorders of water imbalance, there is a unique plasma membrane abnormality in addition to common abnormalities of membrane lipids and proteins, or these patients may differ from the others in their ability to protect against a specific membrane abnormality. Red blood cells and lymphocytes are replaced often; therefore these cells can be useful to follow progressive changes following onset of polydipsia, whereas fibroblasts can be useful to investigate the molecular basis of the core pathophysiology underlying the syndrome. Likely candidates for investigation are the generalized mechanisms of receptor regulation. The role of abnormal lipid metabolism in regulation of receptor functions in fibroblasts from patients with and without water imbalance also can be investigated. Once the structural and functional alterations of plasma membranes and the underlying regulatory processes are investigated in fibroblasts from schizophrenic patients, the molecular biology associated with cellular regulation of water balance also can be addressed.

Therapeutic Possibilities

The therapeutic possibilities will be extensively discussed in other chapters on management of polydipsia and the pharmacology of polydipsia and self-induced dilutional hyponatremia. In this chapter, we discuss the role of cell plasma membrane in regulation of salt and water transport and in receptor-mediated processes that are involved in osmoregulation and AVP regulation of kidney function; therefore, some treatment strategies that involve correcting or protecting cell plasma membranes can be discussed.

The possible developmental membrane deficits associated with polydipsia and cellular membrane pathophysiology underlying the complications of water intoxication indicate that the neuroprotective strategies should be considered. If, for example, ω-3 deficiency early during development is an important factor, it seems unlikely that dietary supplementation of ω-3 fatty acid will be helpful after the syndrome had developed in the adult. However, fatty acid supplementation at critical stages of development may protect against membrane abnormalities that adversely influence the brain development and maturation. Fatty acid abnormalities may occur also from loss by increased lipid peroxidation as a consequence of antioxidant deregulation in schizophrenia (Lohr et al. 1990; Reddy et al. 1991) or by progressive changes owing to water intoxication. These abnormalities may be protected by vitamin E. A developmental deficiency may also be protected by trophic factors, such as growth factors and gangliosides. Growth factors have been found to be neuroprotective against a variety of cell insults (Varon et al. 1988). Gangliosides, a group of naturally occurring compounds that are present in the highest concentrations in neural plasma membranes have been considered to play a critical role in brain and behavior development and in synaptic transmission (Mahadik and Karpiak 1988) and protect against developmental insults (e.g., hypoxia, alcohol, or cocaine) and neural dysfunction as a result of neural injuries in adults (Mahadik 1992; Mahadik and Karpiak 1988).

Chapter 5

Pathophysiology of Fluid Balance Dysregulation in Psychiatric Patients

Morris B. Goldman, M.D.

S ixty years of research into the mechanism of water intoxication in schizophrenia has focused on regulation of water intake, renal water excretion, and vasopressin secretion. Defects in each of these three areas have been characterized, and their relationship to the underlying psychiatric illness and its treatment has been partly clarified. Polydipsia is the most conspicuous abnormality; however, it alone is insufficient to account for hyponatremia, because intake appears to be almost always below levels needed to overwhelm renal diluting capacity (i.e., 25 L/day). Indeed, many schizophrenic patients drink similar amounts of water without any evidence of hyponatremia. Similarly, the defects in renal water excretion, together with the polydipsia, can explain the chronic mild to moderate hyponatremia in the hyponatremic subgroup but not the profound hyponatremia of water intoxication. This effect likely involves transient increases in vasopressin secretion.

FLUID INTAKE

After Hoskins and Sleeper (1933) had identified that urine output was, on average, twice normal in chronic schizophrenic males, the group demonstrated that these patients had no clear impairments in renal or neurohypophyseal function. In particular, their ability to concentrate and dilute urine and directly respond to pituitrin

109

appeared to be normal (Sleeper 1935). Thus, the investigators concluded that the polydipsia was primary and resided "more in the psychical than in the physiological or biochemical domain" (Sleeper and Jellinek 1936).

Since then, the understanding of the physiological regulation of water intake has greatly increased (Grossman 1990; see Chapter 3) but has not been applied extensively to schizophrenic patients. Osmotic regulation of thirst was assessed in one study by measuring the response of polydipsic-hyponatremic and matched nonpolydipsic-normonatremic schizophrenic patients to a standard oral water load (20 ml/kg) and infusion of hypertonic saline (0.1 ml/kg/minute of 3% saline) (M.B. Goldman et al. 1988). At 30-minute intervals during the water load, and 15-minute intervals during the saline infusion, subjects were shown a cup of water and asked how much they wanted to drink. The measure appeared to be valid, because ad libitum intake at the end of the study was significantly correlated to the amount of water desired at that time.

As plasma osmolality increased, desire for water increased in both groups, but levels were consistently higher in the hyponatremic subjects (Figure 5–1). When analysis was restricted to those subjects who were less emotionally withdrawn (as assessed by the Abrams and Taylor scale), the precision (i.e., regression coefficient) and sensitivity (i.e., slope) of the relationship between desire for water and plasma osmolality was similar in the two groups (about one cup for every 5 mOsm/kg increase), but the threshold (i.e., estimated plasma osmolality at which desire for water was zero) was about 10 mOsm/kg lower in the polydipsic-hyponatremic subjects. This leftward shift in the relationship between desire for water and plasma osmolality is similar to that seen in nonpsychiatric patients with compulsive water drinking (Thompson et al. 1991).

These data suggest that osmotic influences on thirst are intact in polydipsic schizophrenic patients but that these patients experience desire for water at lower levels of plasma osmolality. No known or putative factors can account for this difference.

In the only study of the other major physiological regulatory system, the oropharyngeal, four groups were studied: hyponatremic-

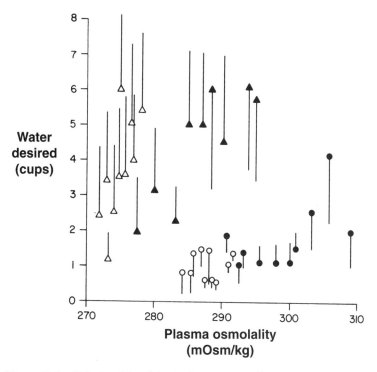

Figure 5–1. Relationship of desire for water to plasma osmolality. Each symbol shows the mean (+ SEM) amount of water desired as a function of mean plasma osmolality at various time intervals during a water load (open symbols) and hypertonic saline infusion (filled symbols). Hyponatremic-polydipsic subjects are represented by circles and normonatremic nonpolydipsic subjects, by triangles.

polydipsic schizophrenic patients, normonatremic-polydipsic schizophrenic patients, normonatremic-nonpolydipsic schizophrenic patients, and normonatremic-nonpolydipsic subjects who were not schizophrenic. Subjects first received an infusion of hypertonic saline (0.1 ml/kg/minute of 3%) for 2 hours to stimulate thirst. Thirty minutes later, subjects were given a 10 ml/kg water load to drink over 5 minutes. Desire for water was determined 15 and 5 minutes before the water load and then every 5 minutes for the next half hour. Desire for water at the end of the study again significantly correlated with actual intake across subjects.

Plasma osmolality after the saline infusion was similar in the three normonatremic groups but was about 10 mOsm/kg lower in the hyponatremic subjects (Figure 5–2). Basal levels of desire for water appeared to differ in the four groups, but as a result of significant individual variation within the groups, the differences were not significant. All four groups showed a significant acute fall in desire for water after the water load. The extent of the fall did not differ between groups; however, levels rapidly rebounded in the two polydipsic groups (Figure 5–2). Although differences in baseline measures and the subjective nature of the scale make it difficult to exclude more subtle defects, these data suggest that the immediate oropharyngeal suppression of thirst is not impaired in polydipsia patients but that this normal response is short-lived. This pattern differs from that in nonpsychiatric patients with compulsive water drinking who show only a minimal drop in thirst immediately after water loading (Thompson et al. 1991). The pattern is consistent, however, with behavioral observations that reveal that polydipsic schizophrenic patients drink similar amounts and report similar levels of satiety as nonpolydipsic schizophrenic patients, but they drink much more often (Shutty et al. 1994).

What these data do not reveal is whether these differences in the regulation of thirst in polydipsic versus nonpolydipsic schizophrenic patients (and nonschizophrenic persons) are a consequence of a defect in thirst regulation or of an unknown factor impinging on an intact regulatory system (Thompson and Baylis 1988). Some believe that thirst regulation per se, is impaired, perhaps by disruption of angiotensin regulation (Verghese et al. 1993). Others attribute polydipsia to hydrophillic delusions or pharmacotherapy acting on intact thirst pathways. Neither of these latter explanations, however, is likely because hydrophillic delusions are rarely endorsed (Millson et al. 1992) and the incidence and severity of polydipsia has not changed significantly with the introduction of modern psychotropic agents (Hoskin 1933; Lawson et al. 1985). Other behaviors associated with schizophrenia, such as compulsions, also appear unable to explain the polydipsia (M.B. Goldman

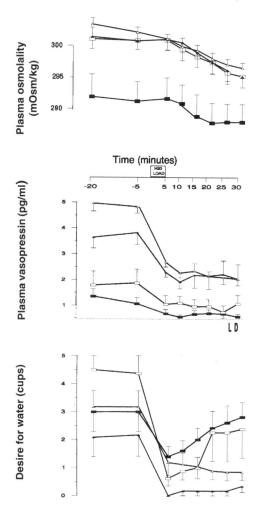

Figure 5–2. Acute effects of oral water loading on plasma vasopressin, desire for water, and plasma osmolality. Each symbol shows the mean (+ SEM) for each variable at a different time interval after an oral water load in patients with hyponatremia and polydipsia (filled squares), normonatremia and polydipsia (open squares), normonatremia and nonpolydipsia (filled triangles), and in control group subjects (open triangles).

and Janecek, 1991). In fact, the relationship between severity of psychiatric symptoms and polydipsia is unclear (Illowsky and Kirch 1988).

A few clues point to areas for further investigation. Most polydipsic schizophrenic patients do not complain of thirst (Hariprasad et al. 1980) but state that drinking relieves some dysphoric state (Millson et al. 1992), and many have a prior history of alcohol abuse, suggesting that the two behaviors may be linked (Ripley et al. 1989). Alternatively, the polydipsia often does not occur until 5 to 10 years after the onset of psychosis, suggesting that it is related to progression of the psychiatric illness (Vieweg et al. 1984b). Another clue is that polydipsia may be associated with excessive repetitive behaviors that are linked to hippocampal dysfunction and dopaminergic activity (Luchins 1990; Luchins et al. 1992; Shutty et al. 1994). Finally, the atypical neuroleptic clozapine (C.M. Canuso and Goldman, unpublished data, April 1995; Leadbetter et al. 1994) diminishes polydipsia and thus may provide a means of clarifying the pathophysiology of the disorder.

In summary, the etiology and mechanism of the polydipsia in schizophrenic patients is unknown, although it cannot be attributed to peripheral stimuli, hydrophillic delusions, or drug therapy. Thirst regulation is altered in these patients, but it is unclear whether this is because of a disruption of thirst or an unknown factor acting on an intact regulatory system. Future studies are needed to

- assess the physiological regulation of thirst in schizophrenia and how it is influenced by acute exacerbations and chronic mental deterioration;
- clarify the internal state that polydipsic patients associate with drinking;
- determine the relationship between polydipsia and this internal state, the severity of the mental disorder, and events in the environment (Shutty et al. 1994);
- clarify the pharmacological profile of "anti-polydipsic agents" and their effect on other aspects of schizophrenia; and
- develop and test animal models to further explore the neuropathology of the disorder (Luchins 1990).

RENAL WATER EXCRETION

In addition to increased fluid intake, about one-fourth of polydipsic schizophrenic patients exhibit mild impairments in renal water excretion (M. B. Goldman et al. 1988). These patients, when stabilized on psychiatric medications, can probably achieve the same degree of urine dilution and water excretion as other schizophrenic patients (and nonschizophrenic patients), but only if plasma osmolality drops to levels well below normal (M.B. Goldman [in press] a). This abnormality, in association with the polydipsia, can account for these patients' basal hyponatremia (i.e., 125–130 mEq/L) but not their episodic water intoxication. Some researchers have failed to identify this impairment (Delva et al. 1990), but these investigators did not systematically alter plasma osmolality nor did they collect sufficient urine samples.

The standard method for assessing renal diluting capacity is to obtain serial urine samples (e.g., every 30 minutes) after an oral water load. In two separate studies, we have found that hyponatremic-polydipsic schizophrenic patients begin to concentrate their urine at lower levels of plasma osmolality than other schizophrenic patients or control subjects (M.B. Goldman et al. 1988, [in press] a). In our recent study with stabilized hyponatremic-polydipsic patients, normonatremic-polydipsic patients, normonatremic-nonpolydipsic subjects, and a control group, we found that the relationship between free water clearance and plasma osmolality was similar in the three normonatremic groups and was decreased in the hyponatremic patients (M. B. Goldman et al. [in press] a) (Figure 5–3). This shift cannot be explained by differences in solute or fluid delivery to diluting segments of the nephron nor can it be attributed to elevated levels of vasopressin or other agents with putative antidiuretic activity (e.g., prolactin or oxytocin) (M. B. Goldman et al. 1988, [in press] a). Furthermore, polydipsia, per se, is an unlikely explanation because the severity of polydipsia appeared to be as great (about 8 L/day) in the normonatremic-polydipsic subjects.

Neuroleptics, however, may enhance the antidiuretic effect of vasopressin (Mitsui et al. 1992), and indeed higher doses of neuroleptics do appear to slightly, but significantly, impair water

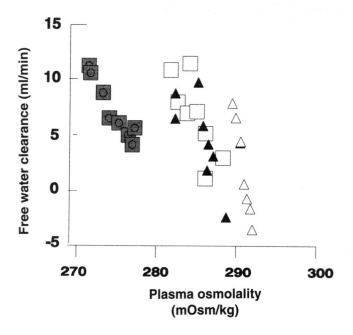

Figure 5–3. Relation of free water clearance to plasma osmolality during water loading. Each symbol shows the mean free water clearance as a function of concurrent mean plasma osmolality. See Figure 5–2 for explanation of the symbols.

excreting capacity (M. B. Goldman et al. [in press] a). Because neuroleptic exposure appears similar in hyponatremic and normonatremic patients, this explanation alone is probably not sufficient to account for the abnormality (M. B. Goldman et al. 1988, [in press] a; Jos et al. 1985). Renal sensitivity to vasopressin could be enhanced by other means. Most intriguing is the possibility of fundamental changes in vasopressin responsivity in the kidney and other areas (e.g., limbic system) that might account for the renal defect and cognitive symptoms of schizophrenia (Bujis 1987). Finally, the sensitivity of vasopressin action and secretion appear to be yoked by an unknown mechanism (e.g., carbamazepine increases and lithium diminishes vasopressin activity, but each has the opposite effect on vasopressin secretion) (Robertson 1987), and alterations of this mechanism might theoretically account for defects in vasopressin action and secretion.

In summary, the diminished renal water excretion is characterized by a lowering of the plasma osmolality required to achieve a given degree of water excretion. Neuroleptics may play some role, although they cannot entirely account for the abnormality. Future studies are needed to 1) clarify whether the defect is present at onset of the psychiatric illness (Emsley et al. 1989) and if, once present, it is relatively stable; and 2) determine whether these patients' kidneys and other sites are hypersensitive to vasopressin.

SECRETION OF VASOPRESSIN

As noted above, the previously identified defects in water intake and renal water excretion are inadequate to account for episodic water intoxication in polydipsic-hyponatremic schizophrenic patients. Many reports show that vasopressin levels are transiently elevated during water intoxication, although it is unclear whether this accounts for all, or even most, of the episodes. It is particularly intriguing that these elevations have been associated with worsening of psychosis and that they frequently resolve with remission of the psychiatric disorder (Riggs et al. 1991; Suzuki et al. 1992).

The latter observation is consistent with studies showing that, when stabilized on optimal doses of antipsychotics, neither the oropharyngeal nor osmotic regulation of vasopressin appear to differ between polydipsic schizophrenic patients with, versus without, a history of hyponatremia. Oropharyngeal regulation of vasopressin was assessed, along with that of desire for water, in the study described above (M. B. Goldman et al. [in press] b). Psychiatric subjects were stabilized on a research unit for 2 weeks prior to the study, and all were treated with fluphenazine. Baseline vasopressin and plasma osmolality were different in the four groups (Figure 5–2). Each group demonstrated the expected acute fall in vasopressin with water drinking, and levels remained suppressed for the remainder of the study. Although the baseline differences again make it difficult to exclude more subtle defects, the response of the hyponatremic subjects was not significantly different from that of normonatremic subjects and suggests this system functions normally, at least when patients are optimally treated and stable.

Osmotic regulation of vasopressin was assessed, following a similar period of stabilization, with a standard oral water load and hypertonic saline infusion (M. B. Goldman et al. [in press]a). When the four groups were compared over a common range of plasma osmolality, all groups showed a significant relationship between plasma vasopressin and plasma osmolality (Figure 5–4). The slope and the intercept appeared to be similar in the two polydipsic groups and less than that of the two nonpolydipsic groups, which also resembled each other. Vasopressin levels for a given plasma osmolality tended to be lower in the polydipsic subjects. Thus, when treated with optimal doses of medication and psychiatrically stable, osmoregulation is not different in polydipsic schizophrenic patients with or without hyponatremia. Osmoregulation appears slightly blunted in both polydipsic groups for unknown reasons. This finding differs from our previous report (M. B. Goldman et al. 1988) and those of other investigators (Delva et al. 1990; Hamozoe et al. 1986; Kishimoto et al. 1989; Saria and Matsunga 1989; Vieweg et al. 1987b) who found that vasopressin levels were consistently higher in hyponatremic subjects. We believe that these differences across studies can be attributed to differences in acclimation to the experimental setting or acuteness of the psychosis (Ragavan et al. 1984).

Heightened vasopressin secretion during psychotic exacerbations, which normalizes with optimal treatment and stabilization of the psychiatric disorder, has been reported with nonpolydipsic schizophrenic patients as well (Emsley et al. 1989; Raskind et al. 1978, 1987). In both instances the mechanism is unclear, and in particular, the role of known (e.g., orthostatic hypotension, cigarette smoking) (Allon et al. 1990) and putative vasopressin stimuli (e.g., neuroleptic treatment) (Ajlouni et al. 1974) have not been assessed. Some researchers believe that the psychotic exacerbation and elevated vasopressin are a cause, rather than a consequence, of the hyponatremia (Inoue et al. 1985).

To clarify the effect of psychotic exacerbations on vasopressin secretion we induced transient exacerbations with the psychotomimetic, methylphenidate. Subjects were matched with polydipsic schizophrenic patients with and without a history of severe

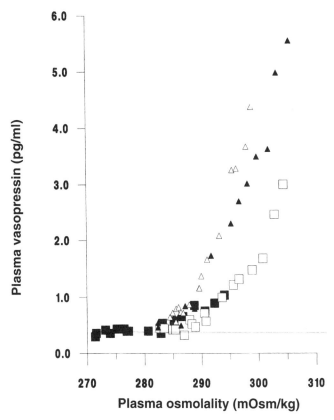

Figure 5–4. Relation of plasma vasopressin level to plasma osmolality during water loading and infusion of hypertonic saline. Each symbol shows the mean plasma osmolality during water loading and the infusion of hypertonic saline. "Common range" (dotted line) marks the range of osmolality used to compare osmoregulation between the four groups. See Figure 5–2 for explanation of symbols.

hyponatremia. The schizophrenic patients were stabilized on the research unit with fluphenazine for 3 weeks prior to receiving intravenous methylphenidate (0.5 mg/kg body weight over 60 seconds), following which blood samples were obtained every

15 minutes for 2 hours. Basal vasopressin levels were near the lower limit of detection of the assay in both groups, and total psychiatric symptoms (as assessed by the Brief Psychiatric Rating Scale) did not differ. Basal plasma osmolality was lower in the hyponatremic patients. Following methylphenidate both groups experienced similar psychotic exacerbations. As expected those subjects with higher plasma osmolalities appeared to have higher peak vasopressin in each group, but the relationship was decreased in the hyponatremic patients (Figure 5–5).

The mechanism of this difference in vasopressin responsivity to acute psychotic exacerbation is unclear. No known vasopressin stimuli could account for the difference. Because osmotic and oropharyngeal regulation appear similar in the two groups, generalized enhancement of vasopressin responsivity is not a viable explanation. Neither is it likely to be a direct consequence of the renal impairment, because this would have been expected to have the opposite effect (i.e., diminished release) (Robertson 1987). Use of neuroleptics and drug-induced dopaminergic hypersensitivity are unlikely explanations because neuroleptic exposure appeared to be similar in the two groups and no subject had clear evidence of tardive dyskinesia prior to or following methylphenidate (M. B. Goldman et al. [in press] a; Illowsky and Kirch 1988; Jos et al. 1985). Stress per se seems untenable, because it does not appear to increase vasopressin in control subjects or nonpsychotic acutely ill psychiatric patients (Edelson and Robertson 1986; Gibbs 1984; Raskind et al. 1978; Wittert et al. 1992).

Thus, an unknown factor likely accounts for this difference. Vasopressin release is modulated by processes acting on axon terminals of the magnocellular neurons, on the dendrites of the magnocellular and adjacent neurons in the hypothalamus, and on the various excitatory or inhibitory pathways scattered through the central nervous system (Morris et al. 1987). Enhanced secretion could be a consequence of differences in releasable vasopressin at the axon terminal or in the activity of a neurotransmitter or neuromodulator, which locally influences release (Sladek and Armstrong 1987). Scattered reports of hypothalamic pathology in schizophrenia (Clardy et al. 1994) and the finding that these patients show abnormal vasopressin response to urea (Ragavan 1984) suggest that this area of the

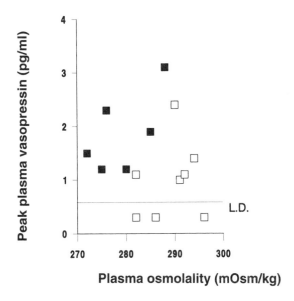

Figure 5–5. Relation of peak plasma vasopressin to plasma osmolality following the psychotimimetic, methylphenidate. Each symbol shows the peak plasma vasopressin and concurrent plasma osmolality in a hyponatremic-polydipsic schizophrenic patient (filled symbol) or a normonatremic polydipsic schizophrenic patient (open symbol).

brain might be implicated in altered vasopressin release. Finally, individual inhibitory or stimulatory pathways might be affected. Of potential interest is the pathway, whose function and associated neurotransmitters are unknown, that projects from the anterior medial temporal lobe to the magnocellular and adjacent neurons of the paraventricular nucleus (Morris et al. 1987). The medial temporal lobe has been implicated in schizophrenia, and evidence of structural impairment is particularly prominent in those with hyponatremia (Kirch et al. 1992). Furthermore, hippocampal lesions in rats appear to enhance the vasopressin response to stress, without enhancing osmoregulation of the hormone (Goldman et al. 1994). Vasopressin appears to be a prominent neurotransmitter in pathways leading back from the neurohypophysis to the medial temporal lobe, and it has been postulated to modulate behaviors and cognitive functions implicated in schizophrenia (Bujis 1987; Winslow et al. 1993). Thus changes to either limb of this pathway theoretically might contribute to enhanced vasopressin release and signs and symptoms of schizophrenia.

In summary, enhanced vasopressin response to psychotic exacerbations appears likely to account for at least some of the episodes of acute water intoxication in polydipsic-hyponatremic schizophrenic patients. No known factors can explain this enhanced release. Future studies are needed to

- determine, as Figure 5–5 suggests, whether psychotic exacerbations enhance vasopressin release in all schizophrenic patients and whether this response resists osmotic suppression in hyponatremic subjects,
- establish whether the osmotic and nonosmotic regulation of vasopressin in hyponatremic schizophrenic patients varies with acuteness of psychiatric symptoms or acclimation to the experimental setting,
- determine whether the vasopressin response to stress per se is enhanced in hyponatremic schizophrenic patients, and
- explore the regulation of vasopressin by the medial temporal lobe and whether disruption of this pathway can induce changes that mimic the physiological and behavioral abnormalities of hyponatremic schizophrenic patients.

CONCLUSION

Interest in the pathophysiology of disordered water balance in psychiatric patients stems from the clinical importance of the disorders, the likelihood these disorders may be traced to defects in known neuroendocrine systems, and the possibility that these defects may provide fundamental insights into the pathophysiology of psychosis. The data suggest that these abnormalities in water balance are not attributable to known pathophysiological mechanisms and thus hold open the possibility that further investigations may lead to important new knowledge. Although water balance does not appear to be fundamentally altered in schizophrenia (with the possible exception of the vasopressin response to psychotic exacerbations), schizophrenia is almost certainly heterogeneous, and the possibility that hyponatremic schizophrenic patients share a common pathophysiology warrants pursuit.

Chapter 6

Structural Brain Imaging in Patients With Schizophrenia and Polydipsia-Hyponatremia Syndrome

Ahmed M. Elkashef, M.D., Robert A. Leadbetter, M.D., and Darrell G. Kirch, M.D.

L ong before neuroleptic medications were introduced for the treatment of psychosis, there was evidence that a significant number of chronically ill psychiatric patients were polydipsic, having increased water consumption and urine output (Lawson et al. 1985; Sleeper and Jellinek 1936). Although this syndrome, as well as its potential for concomitant morbidity and mortality, is now more widely recognized (Lawson et al. 1985; Vieweg et al. 1984a), its etiology remains unknown. Similarly, it is unclear whether any specific central nervous system pathology is associated with poly-dipsia-hyponatremia syndrome.

In this chapter, we review brain-imaging studies that address whether schizophrenic patients with polydipsia-hyponatremia syndrome have structural brain abnormalities that distinguish them from schizophrenic patients without water imbalance and from individuals with no psychiatric or water balance disorders. First a brief overview of the structural neuropathology reported to be associated with schizophrenia in general is presented, and then studies focusing on the subgroup of schizophrenic patients with polydipsia-hyponatremia syndrome are discussed. The possible implications of these findings for the pathophysiology of water imbalance in schizophrenia are outlined, and the potential applications of advancing brain-imaging techniques to the study of this problem are addressed.

NEUROPATHOLOGICAL AND STRUCTURAL BRAIN-IMAGING STUDIES

Since Kraepelin (1919) first described the syndrome of dementia praecox in the late 19th century, a series of investigators have searched for structural brain abnormalities in patients with schizophrenia. Initially these studies applied classical neuropathological techniques to the study of postmortem brain tissue.

Postmortem Studies

Results from these studies varied depending on a variety of factors: the anatomical region of interest, changes resulting from agonal and postmortem events, methodological factors causing technical artifacts, and the quality of clinical information.

The cerebral cortex has received the most attention in neuropathological studies of schizophrenia. Meynert (1884) and Alzheimer (1897) reported atrophy of the frontal lobes and cytoarchitectural disruption in deeper layers of the cortex of schizophrenic patients. Early studies by Southard (1915) found similar cortical lesions that tended to involve the left temporal lobe. Since then, many investigators have reported differing degrees of cortical atrophy in patients with schizophrenia (Andreasen et al. 1986; Kirch and Weinberger 1986). However, the location and type of reported neuropathological changes have been inconsistent, with no identification of a pathognomonic lesion.

Subcortical basal ganglia neuropathological findings have also been reported in postmortem studies since the early 1920s. Cellular alterations such as focal cell loss, sclerotic changes, and dwarf cells have been described in the globus pallidus (Casanova et al. 1992). Decreased volume of the nucleus accumbens and the internal globus pallidus have also been reported (Bogerts et al. 1985). In contrast, bilaterally increased striatal and globus pallidi volumes have been identified in a more recent postmortem study (Heckers et al. 1991).

Limbic system pathology has been reported in multiple post-mortem studies of schizophrenic patients. Smaller volumes in the amygdala and hippocampal formation were cited in several studies (Bogerts 1984; Bogerts et al. 1985, 1993). Smaller parahippocampal gyrus volume was also reported in another study (Altshuler et al. 1990). A decreased number of pyramidal cells in the hippocampus (Falkai and Bogerts 1986; Jeste and Lohr 1989) and disorientation of hippocampal pyramidal cells (Scheibel and Kovelman 1981) also support presumed limbic pathology.

Computed Tomographic Studies

Since the late 1970s and throughout the 1980s, computed tomographic (CT) brain-imaging techniques have been applied to schizophrenic patients. It is interesting to note that earlier pneumoencephalographic studies by Jacobi and Winkler (1927) found lateral ventricular enlargement in patients with schizophrenia. This finding long predated the CT studies in which ventricular size was consistently found to be increased in both the lateral and the third ventricles and, to a lesser extent, cortical atrophy was evidenced by widened cortical sulci (Shelton and Weinberger 1986). Subsequently, patients with schizophrenia were reported to have an increased ventricular-to-brain ratio (VBR) compared with control subjects. The cortical atrophy in most studies was described as global. In 14 studies where regional measurements of sulci were made, no difference was found between anterior–posterior or left to right sulci (Raz and Raz 1990).

Magnetic Resonance Imaging Studies

The advent of magnetic resonance imaging (MRI), which offers many advantages over CT, has revolutionized the field of brain imaging. Because MRI uses electromagnetic energy with little exposure risk compared with the use of ionizing radiation in CT, it allows for longitudinal studies with frequent scanning. In addition, MRI provides excellent soft-tissue rendition, with very high gray–white matter distinction, and it offers great flexibility in plane imaging and in slice thickness. Coronal, sagittal, and axial slices are all possible. Finally, major sulci and temporal regions can be visualized in detail with MRI.

Numerous MRI studies have confirmed earlier CT findings of increased lateral and third ventricular volume in schizophrenia (Gur 1992; Waldman 1992). Although one MRI study of cortical regions in patients with schizophrenia versus control subjects found a smaller frontal lobe area as measured in a single midsagittal slice (Andreasen et al. 1986), Kelsoe et al. (1988) found no differences in prefrontal volumes. More recently, Breier et al. (1992) reported significantly decreased left and right prefrontal volumes in patients with schizophrenia versus control subjects. The temporal lobe and the amygdala-hippocampus have been assessed in several MRI studies with mixed results. Kelsoe et al. (1988) reported no difference in temporal lobe or amygdala-hippocampus volumes, whereas DeLisi et al. (1988) reported a smaller total limbic complex in patients with schizophrenia as measured from a single slice. Smaller volume of the left temporal lobe compared with the right was also reported in patients with schizophrenia (Johnstone et al. 1989), and similar findings were noted by Coffman and Schwarzkopf (1989). In addition, reduced left amygdala and smaller bilateral superior temporal gyri were described in patients with schizophrenia (Barta et al. 1990). More recently, significant reduction of the volumes of left and right amygdala-hippocampus was reported (Breier et al. 1992). Using a different technique to distinguish gray from white matter, Suddath et al. (1989a) reported smaller temporal lobe gray matter volume in patients with schizophrenia. Similarly, Zipursky and Lim (1990) reported reduction of gray matter in all cortical regions measured in patients with schizophrenia. Breier et al. (1992) reported reduction in the prefrontal white matter in patients with schizophrenia versus control subjects.

In studies of monozygotic twins discordant for schizophrenia, both CT (Reveley and Reveley 1982) and MRI studies (Suddath et al. 1990) found that the affected twin had larger ventricles than the unaffected twin. The MRI study by Suddath et al. (1990) also noted that the affected twin had less total gray matter in the left temporal lobe compared with the right and decreased size of both the right and left anterior hippocampi. Similar findings have recently been reported by Breier et al. (1992). Shenton et al. (1992) reported a significant reduction in the volume of gray matter in the left anterior hippocampus, amygdala, left parahippocampal gyrus, and left superior temporal gyrus.

Basal ganglia morphological characteristics also have been examined using MRI. Jernigan et al. (1991) found the lenticular nucleus to be significantly larger in patients with schizophrenia than in normal control subjects. In another study (Swayze et al. 1992), significant enlargement of the right and left putamen and a trend toward enlargement of the caudate were reported in patients with schizophrenia compared with control subjects. Enlargement of the left caudate nucleus also was reported in a recent MRI study (Breier et al. 1992), and enlargement of the right putamen and both right and left globus pallidus was described in patients with schizophrenia compared with control subjects (Elkashef et al. 1994a).

In summary, studies using both neuropathological and neuroradiological techniques have consistently observed central nervous system structural abnormalities associated with schizophrenia. Although they have not identified a pathognomonic lesion, these studies have provided ample evidence that schizophrenia is a disorder in which a developmental anomaly or a degenerative process has affected brain structure.

CLINICAL CORRELATES OF STRUCTURAL BRAIN-IMAGING STUDIES

Several investigators have attempted to relate brain morphological changes in patients with schizophrenia to different demographic and clinical characteristics. For example, increased ventricular size was initially associated with poor neuroleptic response (Weinberger et al. 1980). Increased VBR was also found to correlate positively with the severity of deficit symptoms (Andreasen et al. 1990; Crow 1980; Johnstone et al. 1978). Andreasen et al. (1990) also reported an association between brain atrophy (as evidenced by smaller cerebrum and cranium size) and negative symptoms, whereas Losonczy et al. (1986) found no significant correlation between VBR and symptom profile.

Correlations between VBR and functional impairment or cognitive deficits have been assessed in patients with schizophrenia using various neuropsychological approaches (Donnelly et al. 1980; Golden et al. 1980, 1982; Johnstone et al. 1976). Increased VBR has also been found to be associated with decreased cerebrospinal fluid (CSF) concentrations of homovanillic acid (HVA) (Losonczy et al. 1986), supporting the theory of a hypodopaminergic state in patients with larger ventricles. Cortical atrophy was associated with decreased CSF HVA and dopamine-β-hydroxylase activity in patients with schizophrenia (van Kammen et al. 1983). Also, larger lateral ventricles were found to be significantly correlated with eye-tracking abnormalities (Blackwood et al. 1992).

Temporal lobe structural changes also have been studied in relation to clinical characteristics in patients with schizophrenia. Left superior temporal gyrus volume was found to correlate with the severity of auditory hallucinations (Barta et al. 1990). In another study (Shenton et al. 1992), the volume of the left posterior superior temporal gyrus correlated negatively with the severity of thought disorder. Bogerts et al. (1993) found a strong association between the severity of positive symptoms and reduction in volume of both right and left mesiotemporal structures in patients with schizophrenia.

In addition, the presence of tardive dyskinesia in patients with schizophrenia was associated with smaller basal ganglia structures in CT as well as in MRI studies (Bartels and Themelis 1983; Elkashef et al. 1994a; Mion et al. 1992).

BRAIN IMAGING IN PATIENTS WITH SCHIZOPHRENIA AND POLYDIPSIA-HYPONATREMIA SYNDROME

Surprisingly, there are few imaging studies in patients with schizophrenia and polydipsia-hyponatremia syndrome. Most imaging studies have not investigated the subgroup of patients with schizophrenia accompanied by polydipsia-hyponatremia syndrome for any structural brain abnormalities that would distinguish them from those without polydipsia-hyponatremia syndrome. This lack of studies is surprising when one considers that polydipsia-hyponatremia syndrome has been described since the early 1930s (Hoskins and Sleeper 1933), has a prevalence estimated to range from 6.6% to 17.5%, and is associated with a morbidity and mortality of about 20% of patients with chronic schizophrenia (Illowsky and Kirch 1988; Jose and Perez-Cruet 1979; Vieweg et al. 1985b).

The brain regions involved in regulating thirst mechanisms, as well as fluid and electrolyte balance, include the hypothalamus and the lamina terminalis, which border the third ventricle (Sklar and Schrier 1983). Luchins (1990) has proposed that hippocampal pathology plays a role in the pathogenesis of the bizarre, repetitive behaviors seen in some patients with chronic schizophrenia, including polydipsia, hoarding, pacing, and stereotypies. This theory suggests that the hypothalamus, hippocampus, and ventricular system are primary target areas to investigate using brain-imaging techniques in patients with schizophrenia accompanied by polydipsia-hyponatremia syndrome. However, a literature search revealed only one case report and two CT studies that addressed this question. One pneumoencephalographic study of a patient with schizophrenia and polydipsia-hyponatremia syndrome (Peterson and Marshall 1975) reported an increase in size of the third and the lateral ventricles. Although Kirch et al. (1985) observed increased VBR in six patients with polydipsia-hyponatremia syndrome compared with control subjects, the group mean VBR did not differ significantly from schizophrenia control subjects with no water imbalance. In a CT study of 18 patients with schizophrenia, Lawson et al. (1991) reported that the subgroup of patients with hyponatremia were more likely to show prefrontal atrophy or increased VBR.

Recently, an MRI study was conducted (D. G. Kirch, unpublished data, 1994) that included 19 patients with schizophrenia and polydipsia-hyponatremia syndrome, 19 patients with schizophrenia and normal water balance, and 19 control subjects. Using 0.5-T picker MRI, 1-cm thick contiguous coronal slices were acquired. Patients with schizophrenia and polydipsia-hyponatremia syndrome were found to have significantly larger lateral and third ventricle volumes compared with control subjects. Although the ventricular volumes in the polydipsia-hyponatremia group also were larger than in the schizophrenia control subjects, the difference was not statistically significant. The amygdala-hippocampus was significantly smaller in patients with polydipsia-hyponatremia syndrome compared with both control subjects and schizophrenia patients with no history of water imbalance. Thus, there is emerging evidence that schizophrenia patients with polydipsia-hyponatremia syndrome have greater brain structural pathology, especially in the amygdala-hippocampus, than other schizophrenic patients.

IMAGING STUDIES OF BRAIN CHANGES IN RESPONSE TO WATER LOADING

A key question is whether any structural neuropathology associated with polydipsia-hyponatremia syndrome is a "trait" of the syndrome or "state" related (i.e., an artifact of water loading or hyponatremia). The pathophysiological changes seen in water intoxication have been investigated using different brain-imaging techniques in preclinical studies in patients during water intoxication and in research studies involving a predetermined water-loading paradigm.

Preclinical Imaging Studies

Both MRI and nuclear magnetic resonance (NMR) spectroscopy have been used to study the effects of water intoxication in animals. In one study (Vlajkovic et al. 1986), dogs were intravenously infused with sterile water at a rate of 5 ml/minute while monitoring their central arterial, venous, and CSF pressure. Brain scans were obtained by MRI at baseline and at 8-minute intervals throughout the experiment. The study showed a progressive increase in CSF pressure with a concomitant decrease in local perfusion pressure (the difference between mean arterial pressure and mean CSF pressure). Brain water content was assessed by measuring the signal intensity on the MRI in different gray-matter as well as white-matter regions. Edema was reported to begin in the gray matter of the cerebral cortex and gradually progress to all parts of the brain. After infusion of a water volume corresponding to 10%–14% of body weight, death ensued with transtentorial and transforaminal herniation causing respiratory arrest. Two experiments have used NMR spectroscopy to assess the pathophysiological changes in rat brain tissue resulting from hyponatremia. In one study

(S. Adler and Simplaceanu 1989), brain pH was measured using NMR spectroscopy after acute hyponatremia was induced. A decrease in brain pH was reported in the acute hyponatremic state, which normalized on recovery and correction of the decreased sodium. This decrease suggests that acute hyponatremia impairs the function of sodium and hydrogen exchange in the brain, which could be partially responsible for the changes in mental status observed during water intoxication. Another NMR spectroscopy study (C. L. Fraser et al. 1989) examined the changes in cerebral energy metabolism in an acute hyponatremic state induced in rats by an intraperitoneal injection of arginine vasopressin and water plus dextrose for 3 days. This study also investigated gender differences. Decreased high-energy phosphate generation with an increase in organic phosphate and intracellular acidosis was found in female rats but not in male rats. This finding suggests a marked impairment in Na^+–K^+ pump function in the hyponatremic state and supports clinical data associating morbidity with severe hyponatremia in women (Ayus et al. 1988).

Clinical Studies

Thus far, only three case reports have described neuroradiological findings associated with water intoxication in humans. Berginer et al. (1985) described CT changes in a 52-year-old female patient with acute iatrogenic water intoxication. Clinically she presented with headache, vomiting, restlessness, drowsiness, grand mal seizures, and abnormal neurological signs. Her serum sodium was 114 mEq/L at the time of the CT study, which revealed narrowing of the third ventricle and small lateral ventricles, probably reflecting diffuse brain edema. A postrecovery CT revealed normalization of these findings, and her clinical symptoms resolved. Trabert et al. (1987) described similar changes in a 48-year-old female patient with presenile dementia. She was noted to have decreased size of the lateral and the third ventricles in the water intoxicated state compared with baseline. Lastly, Utzon and Dessau (1991) described a 40-year-old female patient who presented with a seizure and was found on CT scan to have severe cerebral edema. She was noted to have hypotonic polyuria and hyponatremia as a result of polydipsia, apparently related to her attempt to avoid withdrawal symptoms from the termination of benzodiazepine treatment. Interestingly, all three of these case studies involved female patients, which may further support the notion of increased vulnerability to water intoxication in women.

We (Elkashef et al. 1994b) conducted a pilot study using MRI to examine the effects of water intoxication in three patients with schizophrenia. A baseline scan was obtained at 8:00 A.M., and another scan was done after the patient spontaneously engaged in water loading (as evidenced by increased weight and decreased serum sodium). Compared with the baseline MRI scan, the water-loaded scans of all three patients showed a reduction in size of both the lateral ventricles and the third ventricle, with a decrease in VBR probably reflecting brain edema.

Based on these pilot findings, we are currently examining MRI changes during acute water loading in patients with polydipsia-hyponatremia syndrome. Five patients, all with the diagnosis of chronic schizophrenia, have been studied thus far (A. Elkashef, unpublished data, 1994). At the beginning of the 2-day procedure, patients were randomly assigned to either a water-loading protocol (the "wet" state) or normal fluid intake (the "dry" state), the alternate condition occurring on the subsequent day. During water loading, patients were allowed to consume fluids until one or more of three conditions were met: 1) serum sodium of < 130 mEq/L; 2) serum osmolality of < 280 mOsm/L; or 3) body weight gain of $> 7\%$ from the morning baseline weight.

In the initial group of five patients, serum sodium dropped from a mean of 140.8 mEq/L to 128.4 mEq/L in the "wet" state ($t = 8.639$, $df = 4$, $P = 0.001$). The MRI scan in all patients showed a decrease in VBR after water loading. Although there was no relationship of the "dry" serum sodium to the change in VBR, there was a trend toward an association between the VBR change and the "wet" serum sodium ($r = 0.867$, $P = 0.062$). This relationship seemed to occur in a logarithmic fashion, that is, the lower the serum sodium, the greater the degree of decrease in the VBR (1/VBR versus "wet" serum sodium: $r = 0.989$, $P = 0.002$). Using T1 relaxation time calculations obtained by multiple acquisitions, analysis of brain water content thus far has revealed no consistent findings. Analysis of psychiatric, neuropsychological, and endocrine changes are pending.

Although preliminary, these results support our previous findings (Elkashef et al. 1994) and those of the aforementioned case studies, indicating a decrease in VBR in response to acute water loading. This decrease is probably the result of brain edema. Taken together, these initial brain-imaging studies of patients with polydipsia-hyponatremia syndrome indicate that they may have a greater degree of brain structural pathology that is not simply an artifact of water loading.

Central Pontine Myelinolysis

A demyelinating process of the brain may be associated with rapid correction of hyponatremia. It usually affects the pons, but extrapontine locations such as the basal ganglia, thalamus, lateral geniculate body, or cellebellar white matter may also be involved. This process has been called central pontine myelinolysis (CPM), and it is reviewed in detail by Karp in Chapter 9. Recently, multiple MRI studies have documented demyelinating lesions associated with CPM in the brain, as evidenced by areas of signal hyperintensities involving the pons and sometimes the caudate, putamen, or thalamus (Brunner et al. 1988; Dickoff et al. 1988; Morlan et al. 1990). In another case of CPM, changes were seen in the pons on an MRI. These changes resolved on a scan 3 months later as the patient clinically improved (Ragland et al. 1989). The hyperintensities seen on MRI as a reflection of CPM are clearly distinct from the more general periventricular and limbic structural changes associated with polydipsia-hyponatremia syndrome described above.

FUTURE STUDIES

Brain imaging should be an extremely useful tool to investigate central nervous system pathology in patients with polydipsia-hyponatremia syndrome. As reviewed in this chapter, studies are already underway to investigate structural changes. The excellent gray and white matter resolution that MRI provides makes it possible to measure changes in structures that are poorly visualized by CT, such as the hypothalamus and the amygdala-hippocampus, which are of special interest in polydipsia-hyponatremia syndrome. In addition to anatomical information, MRI also can provide information regarding in vivo water content in brain tissue by measuring changes in signal intensity or T1 relaxation time in the regions of interest. A strong correlation between changes in T1 and the water content of brain tissue has been described (MacDonald et al. 1986).

Another technique capable of providing extremely valuable biochemical information about different brain regions is NMR spectroscopy. The technique is in its infancy, but studies have already provided intriguing preliminary information about schizophrenia (Nasrallah 1992; Pettegrew et al. 1991). Clinical studies can be conducted on patients with polydipsia-hyponatremia syndrome using NMR techniques similar to those employed in preclinical studies described above (S. Adler and Simplaceanu 1989; Vlajkovic et al. 1986) and Na-23 NMR (Winkler et al. 1989). This procedure will allow evaluation of the pathophysiological changes that accompany polydipsia-hyponatremia syndrome (e.g., changes in pH, sodium levels, and osmotic concentration). Other neuroimaging techniques, such as positron-emission tomography or single photon emission computed tomography, could also be used to assess blood flow or specific neurotransmitter receptors in different areas of the brain. All these methods are likely to have interesting applications as the study of polydipsia-hyponatremia syndrome in schizophrenia advances.

Chapter 7

Repetitive Behaviors in Chronic Schizophrenia

Daniel J. Luchins, M.D., and Carla Canuso, M.D.

During the past decade, investigators have focused on the significance of positive (e.g., delusions, hallucinations, formal thought disorder) and/or negative symptoms (e.g., blunted affect, lack of motivation, social withdrawal) to the pathophysiology and treatment of schizophrenia (Andreasen 1982; Crow 1980) and have largely ignored a group of symptoms not easily subserved by either category. Although rather heterogeneous, these symptoms can be conceptualized as the dysfunctional repetition of a behavior that under other circumstances is normal.

HISTORICAL OVERVIEW

Descriptions and interpretations of these repetitive behaviors have appeared for years in the schizophrenia literature, although quantitative studies are rare. Perhaps the most exhaustively described are stereotypies and mannerisms.

Kraepelin (1919) wrote detailed clinical accounts of motor behavior seen in both catatonia and other forms of dementia praecox. He defined stereotypy as "the tendency to the instinctive persistence of the same volitional movements.... It shows itself in continuance of the same positions as well as in the repetition of the same movements or actions"(p. 43). In distinction, mannerisms are "morbidly changed forms"(p. 45) or the gross distortion of common activities. Kraepelin believed motor phenomena characterized by persistence

137

were the result of volitional disorder, emerged as the illness progressed, and portended poor prognosis.

Bleuler (1950) found stereotypy to be "one of the most striking manifestations of schizophrenia. . . [found] in every sphere: that of movement, action, posture, speech, writing, drawing, in musical expression, in the thinking, and in the desires of the hallucinating patients"(p.185). These acts are repeated continuously and are often accompanied by verbigeration (i.e., some word or sentence repeated innumerable times regardless of content and without any intention of communication). Bleuler accepted that "there is a tendency for stereotypies to originate directly from the disease process"(p. 351) but maintained "they are symptomatic acts in the Freudian sense; they provide the means of expression for a complex"(p. 456).

One of the few quantitative studies of sterotypies noted their occurrence in 40% of schizophrenic patients but not in affective-disorder patients (Manschreck et al. 1982). Several other repetitive behaviors were described by Arieti (1974) in what he labeled the "preterminal" and "terminal" stages of schizophrenia. In these stages the classical symptoms of schizophrenia are no longer prominent. Rather, patients with end-stage illness lead a vegetative existence. It is from these stages that Arieti describes hoarding, bizarre grooming, and "primitive oral habits"(p. 361).

The preterminal or third stage of schizophrenia generally occurs 5–15 years after the onset of illness and is characterized by severe disintegrating of thought processes. Arieti describes "picking of the skin, pulling out of hair, performance of rhythm in movements, [and] the most common, the hoarding and the self-decorating habits"(p. 352).

Hoarding is the practice of collecting objects, generally of limited size and without practical use. Often patients carry with them the entire collection, and the most regressed patients may use their own body cavities as sites for the hoarded material. Arieti believed hoarding to be quite frequent and studied a series of 64 female patients with this habit. Forty-eight (75%) carried the diagnosis of schizophrenia, suggesting that hoarding is not pathognomonic of advanced schizophrenia, but rather that schizophrenia is the most common condition leading to a state of such regression.

The "self-decorating habit" is also noted in the third stage. This less common, but more obvious behavior consists of the "primitive use of small objects or stains for decoration of one's body. . . without practical or social purposes"(p. 357). According to Arieti, the fourth or terminal stage is the point at which psychology and neurology coalesce. The final phase begins between 7 and 40 years after the onset of illness and commences with a relative increase in motor activity and "primitive" oral behavior including bulimia, tachyphagia, pica, and coprophagia. "Food grabbers"(p. 362) are those patients who cannot prevent themselves from grabbing food at the sight of it. Many such patients go on to develop the habit of placing any object in the mouth, irrespective of edibility (pica).

Arieti attempted to understand many of these unusual behaviors by regarding them as primative habits characteristic of a regressed state analogous to an early phylogenetic stage. Additionally, however, he drew a parallel between characteristic fourth-stage behaviors and those described by Kluver and Bucy (1939) in monkeys with bitemporal extirpation. Such animals showed hyperorality, hypersexuality, hypermetamorphosis, and passivity.

As evidenced by the existence of an entire volume devoted to polydipsia, there has been great interest in this behavior. It is known that polydipsia occurs in about 25% of chronic schizophrenic in-patients, irrespective of medication use (Lawson et al. 1985; Sleeper 1935). Early work on the phenomenon dates back to the 1930s when Hoskins and Sleeper (1933), seeking a physiological basis for schizophrenia, compared the "organic functions" of 92 male inpatients at Worchester State Hospital with nonschizophrenic control subjects. They found the average urinary volume of schizophrenic patients to be twice that of the control group and the individual variability in the pattern of elimination to be three times as great.

Sleeper (1935) subsequently investigated the etiology of this polyuria. Through water load and deprivation trials he was able to demonstrate that the polyuria was secondary to polydipsia and that diabetes insipidus was not present. He also noted that many of the patients in the series who showed a high urinary output had relatively long hospitalizations.

One of the few repetitive behaviors that has been quantitatively investigated in schizophrenia is smoking. Smoking has also been shown to be increased in schizophrenic patients (80%) versus the general population (56%) (Masterson and O'Shea 1984). These repetitive behaviors cause significant morbidity. Polydipsia is associated with protozoal infections, urinary tract dysfunction, pathological fractures, and water intoxication (see M. Goldman 1991 for a review). In many cases, polydipsia and water intoxication are primary reasons a patient cannot be discharged from the hospital. In our clinical experience, bulimia not infrequently leads to death from choking, and pica causes bowel perforation. The sequelae of smoking are well known.

QUANTITATIVE STUDY

Because prior accounts of repetitive behaviors have been mostly descriptive and not quantitative, we recently undertook a study of their prevalence and severity (Luchins et al. 1992a). The study examined 32 chronic schizophrenic patients residing on a 70-bed extended-treatment unit. To assess repetitive behaviors and contrast them to other schizophrenic symptoms, we used the Elgin Behavioral Rating Scale. After reviewing Bleuler (1950) and Arieti (1974) we included eight repetitive behaviors (bizarre grooming, bulimia, hoarding, nicotine-associated behaviors, pacing, pica, and polydipsia). In addition, hypersexuality was added to test Arieti's hypothesis that some patients' behavior was analogous to monkeys with temporal lobectomies. The instrument also included four positive symptoms (hallucinating behavior, suspiciousness, unusual ideas, and disorganized speech) and four negative symptoms (social withdrawal, blunted affect, motor retardation, and depressive mood) drawn from the Psychiatric Symptoms Assessment Scale (Bigelow and Berthot 1989). These positive and negative symptom items were chosen to allow us to compare the severity of repetitive behaviors and the more commonly described schizophrenic symptoms. Items were scored using anchor points on a 7-point scale with 0 denoting none; 1–2, mild; 3–4, moderate; and 5–6, severe symptoms (see Figure 7–1).

Raters assessed patients three times weekly at the end of the shift for symptoms shown during that day and again at the end of the week to generate an overall rating of symptoms seen during the week. Mean weekly ratings were used for all analyses.

The 32 patients (56% female, 59% black) had a mean age of 39 years (SD = ± 9), had a mean of 10.7 years of education (SD = ± 1.6), and had spent a mean total of 16.7 years in the hospital (SD = ± 6.7). Their mean antipsychotic dosage in chlorpromazine equivalents was 538 mg (± 418) (Davis 1974). The mean (± SD) severity of symptoms is presented in Figure 7–1. The mean total score on all eight repetitive behaviors (10.3 ± 6.1) was less than that for the eight positive or negative symptoms (15.3 ± 8.9, *t* = 4.1, *P* = 0.0001). Fifteen of the 32 (47%) patients had at least one severe or two moderate repetitive behaviors, whereas 20 (63%) met this criterion for the positive or negative symptoms. Eleven of the fifteen (73%) who met this criteria for repetitive behaviors also did so for positive and negative symptoms. Although comparison of the severity of different symptoms is problematic, the eight repetitive symptoms appeared to be about two-thirds as prominent as the eight positive or negative symptoms.

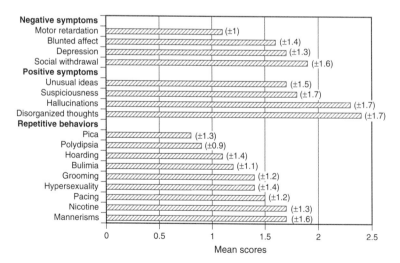

Figure 7–1.   Mean (± SD) global ratings for 32 chronically hospitalized schizophrenic patients on the Elgin Behavioral Rating Scale.

To test the hypothesis that these behaviors are part of a Kluver-Bucy syndrome, we examined the correlation of hypersexuality to oral symptoms. Hypersexuality was significantly correlated only with bulimia ($r = 0.45$, $P = 0.009$), but not with smoking ($r = -0.05$, $P = 0.78$), pica ($r = -0.005$, $P = 0.98$) or polydipsia ($r = 0.10$, $P = 0.60$). This provides little support for Arieti's view that these behaviors are similar to those seen in animals with bilateral, anterior temporal lobe lesions. To examine the relationship of repetitive behaviors with negative and positive symptoms, we correlated the scores of the seven most reliably rated repetitive behaviors with those of the three most reliably rated positive and the three most reliably rated negative symptoms for all 32 patients. The total score for these repetitive behaviors was significantly correlated with that of the positive ($r = .50$, $P = 0.004$) but not of the negative symptoms ($r = 0.27$, $P = 0.1$). A similar analysis was carried out correlating each of the seven repetitive behaviors to the positive and negative symptoms. None of the repetitive behaviors was significantly correlated to the negative symptoms, whereas grooming ($r = 0.6$, $P < 0.001$), hoarding ($r = 0.46$, $P < 0.01$), and pacing ($r = 0.38$, $P < 0.05$) were significantly correlated with the positive symptoms.

We computed the relationship of the patients' demographic and clinical characteristics to the seven most reliably rated repetitive behaviors. Using a backward multiple regression, gender, with a preponderance of symptoms in males, was the strongest correlate ($\beta \supseteq = 0.43$, $P = 0.02$); next was a positive relationship to total length of hospitalization ($\beta \supseteq = 0.38$, $P = 0.03$); and the last significant variable was race, with a preponderance of symptoms among white patients ($\beta \supseteq = 0.38$, $P = 0.03$). Age, education, or antipsychotic dose were not significantly related. A comparable analysis for the three reliable positive symptoms revealed no significant relationships to the demographic and clinical variables. A similar analysis using the three reliable negative symptoms revealed one significant relationship, that with gender (male preponderance, $\beta = 0.40$, $P = 0.04$). The meaning of these findings is unclear, although in schizophrenia, less severe psychopathology has often been associated with being female (Seeman 1988). Repetitive behaviors also were related to increased total length of hospitalization. This finding is consistent with the view of Arieti (1974) and Sleeper (1935) that these symptoms occur in the later stages of schizophrenia and suggests that much lower rates of repetitive behaviors might be found in more acute settings. The fact that repetitive behaviors correlate with positive and not negative symptoms argues against the assumption that they are caused by the deficit state. That 73% of the patients having one severe or two moderate repetitive behaviors also met this criteria for positive and negative symptoms suggests that within the chronically hospitalized population patients with one form of psychopathology generally have the other.

A PATHOPHYSIOLOGICAL MODEL

Although earlier writers speculated on the etiology of repetitive behaviors, considering them to have "Freudian" significance related to "orality" or to bilateral temporal injury, another way to think about the significance of these behaviors is to emphasize similarities to certain behaviors induced in conditioning experiments (Luchins 1990). Polydipsia and the other behaviors being discussed are similar to the "superstitious" stereotypic behavior originally described in food-deprived pigeons placed on brief fixed-interval schedules of food reinforcement (Skinner 1948). Such behaviors are "superstitious" because they have nothing to do with the nature of the reinforcer (i.e., food) or the behavior that must be elicited to receive the reinforcer (i.e., bar pressing), yet they occur in the context of other reward-reinforced behaviors. This phenomenon has been extensively studied by Falk (1961), who referred to it as a *schedule-induced behavior*. In animals, such behaviors include drinking, air licking, wheel running, and aggression (Wallace and Singer 1976). In humans, fixed intervals (FI-5 and FI-60 seconds) of reinforcement can produce polydipsia, increased activity, and bizarre behaviors including "blending Cheezels and Coca Cola and drinking the mixture" or "tearing scrap paper into hundreds of pieces and arranging them in symmetrical patterns" (Wallace et al. 1975, p. 653). One study of schedule-induced behavior in schizophrenic patients noted jumping, pacing, grooming, drinking, and increased verbalization (Kachanoff et al. 1973).

The neurobiology of schedule-induced behavior appears to involve the hippocampus and nucleus accumbens and the neurotransmitter dopamine. Hippocampal lesions in rats facilitate the acquisition of schedule-induced polydipsia (Devenport 1978), whereas 6-OH dopamine lesions of nucleus accumbens (Robbins and Koob 1980), but not prefrontal cortex (Christie et al. 1986), block schedule-induced polydipsia as well as other forms of schedule-induced behavior (Wallace et al. 1983). Hippocampal lesions also facilitate a more general increase in activity in reaction to reward situations. Devenport et al. (1981) described rats with hippocampal lesions that were food deprived and fed the same time each day. As the schedule continued, they developed marked increases in motor behavior and stereotypic movements associated with feeding. Such behaviors were blocked by haloperidol. Interestingly, animals without lesions will develop similar responses (L. D. Devenport, personal communication, July 1989) if made very hungry or given D-amphetamine (Devenport et al. 1981).

Devenport et al. (1981) have interpreted this finding to support the view that the hippocampus normally holds in check superfluous behaviors associated with incentive conditioning and helps selectively associate such conditioning with useful behaviors. The stereotypies seen in these animals (rearing, sniffing, and head bobbing) are associated with dopaminergic activation through the ventral-tegmental pathways to structures such as the nucleus accumbens; they are not the "spatially restricted" sterotypies (biting, licking, sniffing without locomotion) associated with dorsal striatal dopamine (Costall and Naylor 1977). Therefore Devenport et al. (1981) argue that the hippocampus is probably acting on the nucleus accumbens to produce the effect. Because the hippocampus sends primarily excitatory fibers to the nucleus accumbens where ventral-tegmental dopamine is inhibitory, an intact hippocampus would inhibit the effect of dopamine on motor activity. There is anatomical evidence of such a hippocampal input to dopaminergic fibers in the nucleus accumbens (Totterdell and Smith 1989).

The idea that hippocampal lesions may be relevant to schizophrenia was originally proposed by Mednick (1970). In children of schizophrenic mothers who go on to develop schizophrenia, he noted histories of perinatal insult and abnormal galvanic skin responses to a loud noise with decreased latency and lack of habituation. The hippocampus (as well as amygdala and cerebellar, Purjinke, cells) is extremely sensitive to anoxia (Friede 1966), a possible concomitant of perinatal insult, and hipppocampally ablated rats show decreased galvanic skin response latencies (Rabe and Haddad 1969) with poor habituation (Kimble 1968). Mednick's hypothesis has been strengthened by recent autopsy studies that have documented structural and neurochemical abnormalities in temporal regions including the hippocampus and its afferent pathways. The existence of a hippocampal abnormality has now been supported by both neuropathological (see Jeste and Lohr 1989) and MRI studies (Suddath et al. 1990). Perhaps most relevant to the discussion of repetitive behaviors is the observation by Suddath et al. (1989b), who compared 12 schizophrenic patients with histories of polydipsia and hyponatremia with 12 schizophrenic patients without such histories, matched for age, sex, and age of onset, and noted decreased temporal grey matter and smaller hippocampus and amygdala in the former group.

How can we tie all of this together? We would argue that in schizophrenic patients there is a hippocampal abnormality, particularly in the left hemisphere (Flor-Henry 1983; Shenton et al. 1992). This abnormality would interfere with the ability to respond selectively to environmental cues associated with reward or arousal and lead to the development of unselected stereotypical responses or "superstitious behaviors" including drinking, pacing, smoking, odd grooming, and so on. Such symptoms would reflect a failure of the hippocampus to modulate the impact of mesolimbic dopaminergic activity on the nucleus accumbens. Similar to superstitious behaviors in animals, these behaviors could be augmented by increases in drive state or stress (MacLennan and Maier 1983) and by dopaminergic drugs such as amphetamines or reduced by dopamine antagonists such as antipsychotics. It is plausible that the same mechanisms may underlie other schizophrenic symptoms, including the rigid repetitive "superstitious" ideas we know as delusions.

Chapter 8

The Polydipsia-Hyponatremia Syndrome and Cognitive Impairment: Pathophysiological Implications

David B. Schnur, M.D., and Scott Smith, M.A.

At present there is little debate regarding the dire clinical consequences of acute water intoxication, and pathophysiological aspects of this condition have been the subject of fruitful research (Delva et al. 1990; M. B. Goldman et al. 1988) However, the possible role that the mechanism of disturbed water balance may play in our understanding of schizophrenia itself is unclear. There are, nevertheless, several reasons to suspect that such a role may exist. First, disturbances in water balance are widely prevalent in the chronically hospitalized schizophrenic population (Vieweg et al. 1989f), disconfirming the notion that polydipsia-hyponatremia syndrome is merely a physiological curiosity. Second, results from water-loading challenges in schizophrenic patients with relatively short durations of hospitalization who do not exhibit abnormal drinking behavior have raised the possibility that a state of antidiuresis, similar to that associated with water intoxication, may represent a subclinical dysregulation that may be present in the acute schizophrenic population (Emsley et al. 1989). Finally, there is no strong evidence that the syndrome of water intoxication found in schizophrenic patients is an artifact either of neuroleptic treatment or of concomitant medi-

147

cal illnesses (Illowsky and Kirch 1988; Raskind et al. 1987). Such considerations raise the possibility that the mechanisms underlying the polydipsia-hyponatremia syndrome in schizophrenic patients may overlap with those associated with schizophrenia itself. This possibility would be particularly intriguing because the physiological determinants of water imbalance have begun to be elucidated. Moreover, polydipsia can be produced reliably in animals through a variety of experimental manipulations and thus may provide a basis for animal models of behavioral deviations associated with schizophrenia (see Chapters 4 and 7).

In this chapter, we explore the implications that disturbances in water balance may have for the pathophysiology of schizophrenia. Emphasis is placed on the relationship between polydipsia-hyponatremia and cognitive functioning in schizophrenia. Cognitive impairment has been associated both with imbalances in water metabolism and with a variety of dysfunctions said to comprise the defect state, a clinical dimension whose study has provided substantial information on neurobiological alterations that may underlie schizophrenia.

COGNITIVE DYSFUNCTION, SCHIZOPHRENIA, AND THE DEFECT STATE

Defect state symptoms are said to represent "an irreversible component of the pathophysiology of schizophrenia that is characteristic of this disease, even though it is not invariably present, particularly in the early stages of the illness" (Crow 1983, p. 80). Furthermore, it has been proposed that the defect state may represent the core of schizophrenia (Keefe et al. 1987) and thus provide important information on the mechanisms underlying this disorder. For example, it has been reported that defect state probands are more readily categorized as schizophrenic patients according to a variety of diagnostic criteria than other chronic schizophrenic patients and also are more likely to have relatives with a history of schizophrenia and schizophrenia spectrum disorders (Keefe et al. 1987).

Several research groups have presented differing criteria for identifying the defect state, all of which seem to have in common the notion that it is associated with poor outcome. Thus, Crow (1991) writes of the type II syndrome associated with unfavorable prognosis and poor response to neuroleptic treatment and characterized by negative symptoms, intellectual deficits, behavioral deterioration, and dyskinesias. The salience of enduring negative symptoms is emphasized by Carpenter et al. (1991) in their formulation of the deficit state. These workers argue that the deficit state differs from the type II syndrome because the latter focuses on cross-sectional assessments, whereas the criteria for the deficit syndrome require that negative symptoms be present for at least 12 months (Carpenter et al. 1991). Nevertheless, as with the type II syndrome, cognitive impairment on neuropsychological testing has been reported to be more pronounced among deficit-state than nondeficit-state patients (Wagman et al. 1987). Finally the notion of Kraepelinian schizophrenia has been advanced to describe a severe subpopulation that either has been continuously hospitalized for 5 years or is completely dependent on the care of others for food, shelter, and the maintenance of personal hygiene (Keefe et al. 1987).

Although attentional disturbances have been considered a prominent characteristic of schizophrenia at least since the time of Kraepelin, intellectual dysfunction, long known to be a feature of the dementias, was considered to be absent in schizophrenia except in the most severe "terminal cases" (Kraepelin 1971). More recently, however, a greater emphasis has been placed on dementia-like impairments in chronic schizophrenic patients. Crow and Mitchell (1975) examined a large number of chronic schizophrenic inpatients who had been hospitalized for many years. More than half could not state their age correctly. A subgroup distinguished by mannerisms, stereotypic speech, and poverty of speech was particularly incapacitated, identifying their age as being within 5 years of their age at admission despite a 28.4-year mean duration of hospitalization. The authors suggested that age disorientation may identify a specific subpopulation of deteriorated schizophrenic patients who are impaired in their capacity to acquire new information. In a subsequent article appearing 3 years later (Johnstone et al. 1978), this group reexamined 9 of the age-disoriented schizophrenic patients from the previous study, comparing them to 9 age-oriented schizophrenic patients, 10 medical control subjects who had been confined to the hospital for several years, and 8 nonschizophrenic control subjects. Intellectual performance was poorest in the age-disoriented group, but both groups of schizophrenic patients performed worse than either the medical or normal (age and occupation status matched hospital staff) control groups. In addition, impaired intellectual function was associated with negative symptoms and ventricular enlargement on computed tomography (CT) scan. In a more extensive examination of 510 schizophrenic inpatients, Owens and Johnstone (1980) found that the majority showed significant cognitive deficits and that these deficits were related to negative symptoms, movement disorders, and behavioral abnormalities. These deficits were not a result of somatic treatments, but the authors did not measure the contribution of prolonged institutionalization to cognitive impairment.

This latter association was examined in a subsequent article (Johnstone et al. 1981) that compared 120 schizophrenic outpatients to the 510 inpatients previously described. When corrections were made for duration of illness and age, no significant differences emerged between groups in severity of positive or negative symptoms and behavioral disturbance. However, the outpatients exhibited better cognitive performance, although a subgroup of these demonstrated substantial impairments. It was concluded that the deficits observed in schizophrenic patients resulted from the disease and were not an artifact of institutionalization. Cognitive impairment, however, could be worsened by prolonged hospitalization. Alternatively, cognitive impairment might be associated with prolonged hospitalization, because it characterized a treatment refractory patient group (Johnstone et al. 1981). More recently, the relationship between cognitive functioning and duration of hospitalization in a sample of 245 schizophrenic patients was studied by Goldstein et al. (1991) using multiple regression techniques. When age and education were accounted for, duration of hospitalization was not found to contribute significantly to the variance in cognitive test performance.

A somewhat different approach to the question of cognitive functioning has used IQ test results and suggests that schizophrenia is associated with reduced intellectual performance. This evidence, subjected to metaanalysis by Aylward et al. (1984), indicates that schizophrenic patients who are tested after the onset of illness have lower IQ scores than their siblings or control subjects but not when compared with groups with other psychotic disorders. The premorbid IQs of schizophrenic patients appear to be lower than either nonpatient age matched control groups or siblings.

Among schizophrenic patients, low IQ may be associated with early onset of illness and poor outcome, particularly in males. Declines in IQ measured after the onset of illness also may be associated with poor clinical outcome (Aylward et al. 1984). In conformity with this latter view, Heaton and Drexler (1987) found that the cognitive impairment associated with schizophrenia was not caused by somatic treatment and that progressive worsening of neuropsychological test performance may be a feature of patients with poor clinical outcome.

In aggregate, the evidence outlined above suggests that reductions in cognitive performance characterize a substantial proportion of the schizophrenic population and may be demonstrated either by clinical observation or through the use of standardized testing procedures. Neither the side effects of somatic treatment nor institutionalization appears to account for these impairments. Instead, their association with poor outcome and negative symptoms suggests that they are related to the defect state.

COGNITIVE PERFORMANCE AND WATER BALANCE

An early study by Sleeper and Jellinek (1936) is informative because it was carried out before the neuroleptic era. Using an initial sample of 92 male schizophrenic patients on whom urine volumes had been determined (Hoskins and Sleeper 1933), these authors compared the 12 patients with the highest and lowest urine volumes on a number of measures. No differences were noted in age and duration of hospitalization between the two groups. However they found a mean IQ of 92 in the group with high urine volume compared with 73 in the low urine volume group, although these differences did not attain statistical significance. In addition, when a clinical index of "emotional" functioning was examined, it was found that the high urine volume group showed significantly less deterioration. These authors concluded that "the long persistent polyuria in the 'high' [urine volume group] apparently produces no deleterious effects on the body economy" (Sleeper and Jellenek 1936, p. 562).

This study indicates that although polyuria is not an artifact of neuroleptic treatment in schizophrenic patients, it is not associated with the defect state. However, the implications for the polydipsia-hyponatremia syndrome are unclear as neither serum sodium concentration nor osmolality was measured. More recently, Lawson et al. (1985) presented evidence that is congruent with Sleeper and Jellinek (1936), reporting that urine output was positively associated with good premorbid functioning and favorable response to neuroleptics. Measures of serum and urine osmolality and of serum sodium indicated that abnormalities consistent with antidiuretic hormone dysfunction were not present in this sample, although three of seven patients were hyponatremic. The authors suggested that polydipsia without hyponatremia may be associated with the type I dimension of schizophrenia characterized by good outcome and a predominance of positive symptoms (Crow 1991).

By contrast, Kirch et al. (1985) reported evidence that may be consistent with an association between cognitive deterioration and the polydipsia-hyponatremia syndrome. Case reviews were conducted of all patients at Saint Elizabeths Hospital, Washington, D.C., with serum sodium levels that were < 133 mmol/L on at least two occasions during a 3-month period. The authors suggested that a significant proportion of hyponatremic patients without symptoms of water intoxication may not have been examined, because serum sodium was not routinely assessed at the time. After excluding patients in whom hyponatremia may have resulted from medical problems, eight patients (four females) with chronic undifferentiated schizophrenia were identified as having polydipsia-hyponatremia. Of these, four had a history of hyponatremic seizures. Mean IQ for four of the patients was 74.5 (range 70–83). The authors did not indicate which of these patients, if any, had a seizure history. Previous IQ tests carried out 8–20 years earlier were available on three of the patients and indicated that their scores had declined between 15 and 54 points. Although IQ results were not compared with a schizophrenic control group, these results are of interest because others have reported that declines in IQ test performance may be related to poor symptomatic outcome in schizophrenic patients (Aylward et al. 1984). One conclusion of this report was that self-induced dilutional hyponatremia may be associated with Crow's type II dimension.

Recently, we (Schnur et al. 1993) examined the relationship between cognitive functioning indexed by the Mini-Mental State Exam (MMSE)(Folstein et al. 1975) and polydipsia-hyponatremia syndrome. The rationale for the study was provided by Luchins (1990), who suggested that polydipsia and other stereotypic behaviors may be determined by temporal lobe disturbances, specifically by hippocampal dysfunctions that disrupt arousal and responses to stimuli associated with reward (Luchins 1990). Furthermore, it is known that temporal lobe dysfunction is associated with a variety of cognitive deficits and that both structural (Jeste and Lohr 1989) and functional (Gruzelier et al. 1988) temporal lobe disturbances are seen in schizophrenia. Accordingly, we hypothesized that polydipsia-hyponatremia syndrome would be associated with poor performance on the MMSE, possibly as a result of temporal lobe dysfunction.

We were also interested in determining whether cognitive impairments depended on the coexistence of hyponatremia at the time of the cognitive assessments. Vieweg et al. (1984c) had demonstrated that cognitive performance may decline as patients become hyponatremic by examining relations between MMSE scores and serum sodium levels in four schizophrenic patients with polydipsia-hyponatremia syndrome. When the patients were examined as a group, positive correlations between MMSE scores and sodium levels were evident, suggesting that hyponatremia may worsen cognitive functioning. Thus, to provide preliminary evidence that the relationship between the polydipsia-hyponatremia syndrome and cognitive impairment that was not simply a result of the hyponatremic state itself, our study examined intellectual functioning in patients with a history of polydipsia-hyponatremia but with normal serum sodium levels at the time that they were being evaluated.

We compared MMSE scores of 13 schizophrenic patients who had had at least one episode of polydipsia-hyponatremia syndrome with 20 schizophrenic control subjects. The latter group had neither a known history of polydipsia nor of hyponatremia. All of the poly-dipsic-hyponatremic patients had morning blood samples analyzed on the day of the cognitive assessments and were only included if their sodium levels were > 135 mmol/L.

The demographic characteristics of the sample have been presented elsewhere (Schnur et al. 1993). The polydipsic-hyponatremic group had been hospitalized for a significantly longer period of time but did not differ from the control group on other demographic variables. As indicated in Figure 8–1, the polydipsic-hyponatremic patients performed worse on all MMSE items, with differences attaining statistical significance on items for orientation to time, sentence writing, and design copying. In addition, MMSE total scores were significantly less in the patients with the polydipsia-hyponatremia syndrome ($P < 0.01$). A score of 23 or less on the MMSE is considered to indicate significant cognitive impairment (Tombaugh and McIntyre 1992). Using this cutoff, we found that 39% of the total sample exhibited such cognitive impairment. As Figure 8–2 indicates, there was a higher proportion of cognitively impaired patients in the polydipsia-hyponatremia syndrome subsample, but this difference was not statistically significant.

Prolonged stay on an inpatient ward may worsen cognitive functioning in chronic psychiatric patients. This effect may be particularly true of polydipsic patients, many of whom require confinement to the ward under close supervision to prevent excessive consumption of liquids. Indeed, in our sample the length of hospitalization was much greater in the polydipsic-hyponatremic group than in the schizophrenic control group, although there were no differences in duration of illness (Schnur et al. 1993). To examine the contribution of length of hospitalization to MMSE results, we reexamined MMSE total scores after omitting the item pertaining to temporal orientation. This reanalysis was undertaken to establish that poor performance on the MMSE resulted from cognitive weakness rather than from decreased access to time markers in the hospital setting. The results indicated that overall MMSE differences between groups were not caused by disorientation to time. Cognitive performance remained significantly worse in patients with a history of polydipsia-

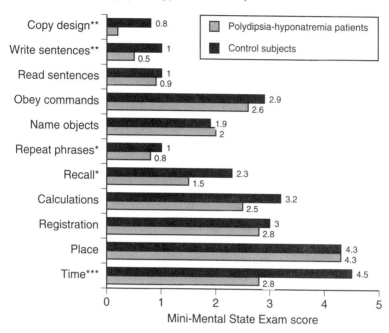

Figure 8–1. Mini-Mental State Exam scores in schizophrenic patients with and without a history of polydipsia-hyponatremia syndrome. The numerals next to the bars refer to the mean values of the corresponding items of the MMSE. *$P < 0.1$; **$P < 0.005$; ***$P < 0.0005$

hyponatremia ($t[11] = -2.2$, P [2-tailed] $= 0.03$). In addition, length of hospitalization was not significantly correlated either to temporal orientation or to MMSE total scores (Pearson $r = -0.27$ and 0.23, respectively, both $P < 0.1$), again suggesting that apparent cognitive impairment was not an artifact of prolonged hospitalization. This result is consistent with the evidence described above that neuropsychological dysfunction in chronic schizophrenic patients cannot be explained by length of hospitalization (G. Goldstein et al. 1991).

It was also important to examine the role that a history of hyponatremic seizures might play in the cognitive performance of our sample. A seizure history might reduce MMSE score for three reasons:

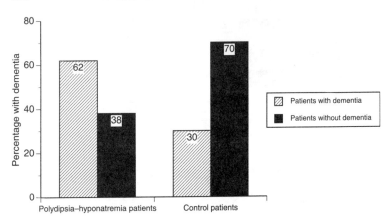

Figure 8–2. Proportions of patients with cognitive impairment. Patients with an MMSE total score of 23 or less were considered to have cognitive impairment comparable to that found in the dementias. Cutoff for cognitive impairment determined from Tombaugh and McIntyre (1992).

1. Such a history might reflect a more severe condition, with more frequent and prolonged episodes of water intoxication that might produce brain damage.
2. The seizures themselves may have been associated with cerebral hypoxia that could be injurious to the brain.
3. The treatment of the seizures may have resulted in brain damage.

It is known that the rapid correction of hyponatremia can cause massive cognitive impairment associated with demyelinating lesions in the pons and extrapontine sites (Tien et al. 1992; Chapter 9). Of the 11 patients with a history of polydipsia-hyponatremia syndrome, five had a history of seizures. When we compared their MMSE performance with that of the polydipsic-hyponatremic patients who had no seizure history, we found no significant differences (t [11] = 0.2, $P < 0.1$). These results do not support the view that the relationship between polydipsia-hyponatremia syndrome and cognitive impairment is attributable to seizures.

Although our study provided initial evidence that the polydipsia-hyponatremia syndrome may be associated with cognitive impairment in patients who have normal serum sodium levels on the day of the cognitive assessment, certain methodological shortcomings may be pertinent. We were unable to carry out all MMSE evaluations in the morning, and it is possible that some of the polydipsic patients who were tested in the afternoon had become hyponatremic by then. Hyponatremia is known to worsen in the afternoon in patients with polydipsia (Koczapski and Millson 1989). However, patients who were actively polydipsic were under close supervision to prevent them from drinking excessively, making this scenario unlikely. It is also possible that the polydipsic patients failed to cooperate with the MMSE because of psychosis. Standardized symptom ratings were not carried out on these patients, but our impression is that the two experimental groups did not differ in severity of psychosis. Furthermore, there were no differences between groups on several of the MMSE items that required patient cooperation, such as obeying commands and sentence reading (Figure 8–1).

Relatively poorer cognitive functioning in schizophrenic patients with disturbed water balance was also reported by Emsley et al. (1993). These workers administered neuropsychological tests to 16 inpatients, consisting of five with polydipsia, five with dilutional hyponatremia and impaired urinary diluting capacity, and six with both conditions. Test performance was compared with a control group of chronic schizophrenic inpatients without a history of water imbalance that was matched for age, gender, educational status, sociodemographic background, and duration of illness. The principal findings were poorer visual memory and visuomotor integration in the group with dysregulated water balance. As with our study, group differences could not be explained by a history of water intoxication because such patients did not perform more poorly on neuropsychological testing than the remainder of the group with water imbalance. Groups did not differ in estimated premorbid IQ, frequency of tardive dyskinesia, or severity of symptomatic state. Specifically, ratings of both positive and negative symptoms using the Positive and Negative Symptom Scale for Schizophrenia (Kay et al. 1987) were similar in the two groups. Serum sodium levels were not measured on the day of the neuropsychological assessments. However, patients were tested in the morning and prevented from drinking before and during the evaluation.

Methodological questions aside, this evidence raises the possibility that polydipsia-hyponatremia and cognitive impairment share in common certain underlying pathogenic mechanisms. Although these mechanisms remain unknown, there is indirect evidence suggesting that structural brain abnormalities may be implicated. It has been proposed on the basis of animal lesion studies that polydipsia represents one of a number of stereotypic behaviors that may be subserved by hippocampal dysfunction (Luchins 1990). Clinical studies in schizophrenic patients have suggested that cognitive impairment may also be associated with mannerisms—the human variant of stereotypy (Crow and Mitchel 1975)—perhaps even more robustly than with negative symptoms (Bilder et al. 1985). Furthermore, although there are inconsistencies, an abundance of evidence suggests that cognitive impairments may be determined by structural brain abnormalities in schizophrenic patients (Shelton and Weinberger 1986). Recent evidence suggests that reductions in the volumes of the amygdala—hippocampal complex-structures that are critical for intellectual functioning—are greater in schizophrenic patients with polydipsia-hyponatremia than schizophrenic control subjects (Chapter 6). Taken together, these findings underscore the need to examine further the relationship between polydipsia-hyponatremia, cognitive impairments, and structural brain abnormalities. Although it is of interest that a formulation by Crow (1985) suggested that the locus for cell loss underlying the type II syndrome may reside in the temporal lobes, the results of the cognitive evaluations performed on polydipsic-hyponatremic patients have not implicated a specific area of the brain.

POLYDIPSIA-HYPONATREMIA SYNDROME AND THE DEFECT STATE

Although the mechanisms of the defect state and polydipsia-hyponatremia syndrome have not yet been elucidated, it is possible that pathophysiological aspects of these two entities may overlap. As indicated in Table 8–1, there are several components of the defect state, in addition to cognitive impairment, that also may be associated with the polydipsia-hyponatremia syndrome. However, the relationship between polydipsia-hyponatremia and the defect state has not been systematically studied, and the relevant research has often been limited by small sample size and the failure to replicate findings. The following discussion, therefore, is being presented for heuristic purposes.

Prolonged Duration of Illness and Length of Hospitalization

It is rare that the defect state is manifest at the onset of the schizophrenic illness. Rather, such deterioration commonly supervenes after the illness has already followed a chronic course. This finding has been illustrated by Pfohl and Winokur (1982) who found that negative symptoms, mannerisms, and cognitive impairment first became evident an average of 5 years after the first hospitalization in contradistinction to hallucinations and delusions that were manifest at the onset of illness. Similarly, the proportion of schizophrenic patients with disturbed water metabolism indexed by excessive diurnal weight gain was greater among more chronic patients when two groups of schizophrenic patients were compared, one with a mean duration of illness of 14.6 years and the other having been ill on average for 3.8 years (Vieweg et al. 1989f). More recently, we have reported that duration of hospitalization is markedly longer in poly-dipsic-hyponatremic patients when compared with schizophrenic control subjects with similar duration of illness, suggesting that the

---

Table 8–1.   Possible "defect state" features of polydipsia-hyponatremia syndrome

1. Cognitive impairment.
2. Prolonged duration of illness and length of hospitalization.
3. Structural brain abnormalities.
4. Tardive dyskinesia
5. Nonsupression of the dexamethasone supression test.
6. Age of onset.

former group is characterized by a more chronic course (Schnur et al. 1993). In contrast, Emsley et al. (1989) reported results of water-loading tests consistent with a state of antidiuresis being present in normonatremic schizophrenic and schizoaffective patients with short lengths of hospitalization. Taken together, these findings might suggest that although full-blown polydipsia-hyponatremia syndrome is associated with poor outcome, subclinical evidence of water imbalance may represent a *forme fruste* of this condition that is not associated with defect-state symptoms.

Structural Brain Abnormalities

Although there are inconsistencies in the literature (Owens et al. 1985), there appears to be agreement by most authors that defect-state symptoms are associated with structural brain abnormalities (S. Olson et al. 1991; Shelton and Weinburger 1986). The neuroanatomical findings pertinent to polydipsia-hyponatremia syndrome have been reviewed in Chapter 6 and indicate that this condition is associated with ventricular dilitation and sulcal prominence that is not dependent on concomitant hyponatremic encephalopathy.

Tardive Dyskinesia

An association between tardive dyskinesia and the defect state has been proposed by Crow (1991). This link is based on comparisons of schizophrenic patients with and without dyskinetic movements, suggesting that the former may have more severe intellectual impairment, negative symptoms, and structural brain abnormalities (Owens et al. 1985; Waddington and Youssef 1986). Furthermore, dyskinetic movements may be an integral feature of the disease process rather than the result of neuroleptic treatment, as such movements have been noted in drug-naive chronic schizophrenic patents (Owens et al. 1982). A relationship between polydipsia-hyponatremia syndrome and tardive dyskinesia was proposed by Kirch et al. (1985), who found that three of eight patients with polydipsia-hyponatremia syndrome had tardive dyskinesia. However, tardive dyskinesia was unrelated to polydipsia-hyponatremia syndrome in two studies that compared schizophrenic patients with disturbed water balance to schizophrenic control subjects (Emsley et al. 1993; Schnur et al. 1993). In a similar vein, Umbricht et al. (1993) reported that clinical indicators of water metabolism impairment were not associated with tardive dyskinesia in a longitudinal study of 68 patients, of whom 81% had a diagnosis of schizophrenia.

Nonsuppression of the Dexamethasone Suppression Test

Post-dexamethasone suppression test cortisol levels have been found to be associated with a number of characteristics of the defect state in schizophrenic patients. These include negative symptoms in mediation-free (Tandon et al. 1991) and neuroleptic-treated patients (Coppen et al. 1983), reductions in positive symptoms (Harris 1985), and poor performance on cognitive assessments (Saffer et al. 1985). In addition, persistent dexamethasone suppression test nonsuppression in neuroleptic-treated schizophrenic patients may predict poor outcome (Tandon et al. 1991). This area of research is inconsistent, however, and methodological reasons for divergent findings have been reviewed by Tandon et al. (1991). Regardless, a recent study (M. B. Goldman et al. 1993a) found that dexamethasone suppression test nonsuppression was associated with polydipsia in schizophrenic patients. Goldman et al. suggested that this association may be determined by hippocampal dysfunction that either results in antidiuretic hormone dysregulation or subserves manneristic repetitive behaviors such as polydipsia. The integrity of the hippocampus is critical for the functioning of the hypothalamic pituitary adrenal axis subserving glucocorticoid regulation (Sapolski and Plotski 1990).

Age at Onset

Early age at onset is considered to be a poor prognostic sign of schizophrenia (DeLisi 1992; Johnstone et al. 1989). Recently Crow (1991) suggested that early age at onset may be associated with clinical features of the defect state and that the early development of schizophrenia may be associated with arrested brain maturation. Kirch et al. (1985) found that the mean age at onset of illness in eight patients with polydipsia-hyponatremia syndrome was 20.7 years and commented that this was "relatively early." We examined the age at onset in the 29 state hospital patients presented previously (Schnur et al. 1993). The mean onset of schizophrenia (± SD) was at 19.1 ± 4.5 years and 20.5 ± 4.5 years for patients with and without polydipsia-hyponatremia syndrome, respectively ($P < 0.1$). Although age at onset was similar in the two groups, our findings do not disconfirm the view that polydipsia-hyponatremia syndrome is associated with early-onset schizophrenia because the onset of illness is extremely difficult to determine retrospectively for methodological reasons (Beiser et al. 1993; DeLisi 1992).

Negative Symptoms

Negative symptoms are thought to compose a major clinical characteristic of the defect state. Only one study has examined relationships between negative symptoms and polydipsia-hyponatremia syndrome and has found no differences between schizophrenic patients with and without disordered water metabolism (Emsley et al. 1993). Further study of this issue is needed.

CONCLUSIONS AND DIRECTIONS FOR FUTURE RESEARCH

It is possible that the relation between polydipsia-hyponatremia syndrome and intellectual impairment in schizophrenic patients may be relevant to the pathophysiology of the schizophrenic defect state. This view is based on evidence that cognitive functioning in schizophrenic patients with a history of polydipsia-hyponatremia syndrome is significantly reduced in comparison to a schizophrenic control sample. This finding does not appear to be caused by a concomitant hyponatremic encephalopathy nor can it be readily explained by brain damage resulting from a history of water intoxication. Instead, we suggest that polydipsia-hyponatremia syndrome may reflect disturbances that are related to mechanisms subserving the defect state. In addition, a number of other features reported to be associated with the defect state also may be present in polydipsia-hyponatremia syndrome (Table 8–1). This evidence is inconsistent, however, and further study of the relationship between these two entities is necessary. Such research also should include the examination of the relationship of polydipsia-hyponatremia syndrome to treatment outcome. Also relevant would be the examination in acute patients of the relationship between outcome indicators and subclinical disturbances in water balance (e.g., as manifested in water-loading challenges; Emsley et al. 1989). In addition, the clinical characteristics of schizophrenic patients with polyuria without hyponatremia should be considered, because this group may be characterized by clinical features that are different from those associated with the polydipsia-hyponatremia syndrome.

Moreover, before more definitive hypotheses may be proposed, a number of methodological considerations must be addressed. Included here are sample size, replication studies, and standardization of assessments.

Finally, the question of diagnostic specificity requires further consideration. In addition to being present in schizophrenia, polydipsia-hyponatremia also has been described in mood-disordered patients and in patients with mental retardation (Chapter 1). The implications of such evidence for the schizophrenic defect state are unclear. Indeed, putative characteristics of the defect state, such as poor response to treatment, a deteriorating course, and structural brain abnormalities, have been reported in mood disorders as well as in schizophrenia (Goodwin and Jamison 1990). It is possible that defect-state symptoms represent a terminal stage of the severe psychiatric disorders that is not necessarily the domain of one particular nosological entity. Similarly, this may hold true for the polydipsia-hyponatremia syndrome, pointing to the need to examine this condition and its relations to the defect state across diagnostic groups.

Chapter 9

Water Intoxication: Neurological Aspects of Acute and Chronic Hyponatremia

Barbara Illowsky Karp, M.D.

Neurological dysfunction resulting from "water intoxication" was first described by Rowntree (1923). He observed that animals given pituitary extract and free water became restless, asthenic, had seizures, and died. The neurological illness was associated with brain edema and was believed to be caused by "a disturbance in osmotic relationships and in salt/water equilibrium of the brain and nervous system" (Rowntree 1923, p. 172). Subsequent animal experimentation and human clinical experience have confirmed that symptoms of water intoxication are caused by fluid and electrolyte changes in the brain induced by plasma hypoosmolality. Sodium is the major determinant of plasma osmolality in most circumstances (Verbalis 1989). Water intoxication is therefore almost always associated with hyponatremia.

The severity of illness in water intoxication depends on both the degree of hyponatremia present and the rate with which hyponatremia develops (Arieff et al. 1976; Sterns 1990). Patients with mild hyponatremia have seizures and loss of consciousness if the serum sodium concentration falls quickly, whereas other patients with profoundly low serum sodium levels are asymptomatic if the hyponatremia develops gradually. Water intoxication can be fatal. Symptoms of water intoxication often are reversed by restoration of normonatremia. Rapid correction of hyponatremia, however, is not always safe.

Central pontine and extrapontine myelinolysis is a neurological disorder characterized pathologically by loss of myelin in the pons and certain extrapontine areas of the brain (Adams et al. 1959). This illness can be fatal or cause permanent neurological dysfunction (Goebel and Herman-Ben Zur 1972; McCormick and Danneel 1967; Sterns et al. 1986). Myelinolysis is caused by the rapid correction of hyponatremia. The physician caring for a hyponatremic patient therefore faces a dilemma: Raising the serum sodium concentration to treat a seriously ill, hyponatremic patient may induce central nervous system myelinolysis.

The proper management of hyponatremia recently has been the subject of substantial controversy (Berl 1990a, 1990b; Cluitmans and Meinders 1990; Sterns 1991). Some researchers, focusing on the danger of seizures and hypoxia that can accompany hyponatremia, recommend rapid correction (Arieff 1986, 1991; Arieff et al. 1992; Ayus et al. 1987). Others, concerned about myelinolysis, advocate gradual correction of hyponatremia (Laureno and Karp 1988; Sterns 1987, 1990).

In this chapter, I discuss the signs, symptoms, and pathophysiology of acute and chronic hyponatremia and of myelinolysis. An approach to treating hyponatremia designed to minimize both morbidity from hyponatremia and the risk of myelinolysis with correction is presented.

HYPONATREMIA

Mild hyponatremia (serum sodium [Na+] between 130 and 135 mEq/L) is common in hospitalized patients. Severe hyponatremia (serum [Na+] < 130 mEq/L) occurs in 1%–6% of hospitalized patients (R. J. Anderson et al. 1985; Flear et al. 1981; P. A. Gross et al. 1987) and is associated with an 8%–33% mortality rate (Ayus et al. 1985; Sterns 1987). In Anderson's study, hyponatremic patients were 60 times more likely to die than normonatremic patients (R. J. Anderson et al. 1985). Death in hyponatremic patients is usually as a result of progression of an underlying illness rather than the hyponatremia itself (R. J. Anderson et al. 1985; Sterns 1987).

Hyponatremia causes a generalized metabolic encephalopathy (Levinsky 1991). Early signs include malaise, headache, and irrita-

bility. Tremor, nausea, vomiting, and diarrhea c
time. Generalized tonic-clonic seizures can pers
tus epilepticus if hyponatremia remains untreal
lethargy can progress to coma. Some patients l
chosis (Burnell and Foster 1972; Santy and Schwartz 1966). __
neurological signs, seen only rarely, include anisocoria, hemiparesis,
and ataxia (Daggett et al. 1982). We recently reviewed the records
of 14 patients with corrected hyponatremia (Karp and Laureno,
1993). During the hyponatremic period prior to treatment, these
patients had, in addition to the signs mentioned above, generalized weakness, low-grade fever, anorexia, myalgias, dizziness, urinary incontinence, hiccups, and slurred speech. There is a large
variation in the severity of symptoms seen at a given sodium level,
but symptoms are likely when the serum [Na+] drops below 125
mEq/L (Arieff et al. 1976; Daggett et al. 1982; Sterns 1987). Patients
with a rapid drop in serum sodium are more severely ill than those
whose hyponatremia develops gradually.

Systemic manifestations of hyponatremia reflect its underlying
cause. For example, patients with sodium depletion and hypovolemia have orthostatic hypotension, loss of skin turgor, or azo-
temia, whereas those with edematous states have peripheral edema
and congestive heart failure (Levinsky 1991).

As in most metabolic encephalopathies, imaging studies of the
brain are usually normal in hyponatremic encephalopathy. The
electroencephalogram may show nonspecific slowing or triphasic
waves indicative of generalized cerebral dysfunction. Routine cerebrospinal fluid (CSF) studies are normal.

BRAIN ADAPTATION TO HYPONATREMIA

Hyponatremia develops when electrolytes are lost or fluid intake
overcomes the body's large capacity for fluid excretion. Impaired
excretion of free water may also be present. Hyponatremia may
occur in severe gastroenteritis with diarrhea and vomiting. It may
follow the infusion of large volumes of hypotonic fluids given intravenously. Fluid administration by other routes such as bladder
irrigation during prostate surgery or proctolysis in patients with
self-administered cleansing regimens may lead to hyponatremia.

Hyponatremia may develop with the administration of oxytocin during gynecological procedures or in patients with diuretic or laxative abuse (Bhagavan et al. 1976; Brunner et al. 1990; Castillo et al. 1989; Copeland 1989; D. Fraser, 1988; Gerard et al. 1987; Greenberg et al. 1992; Ragland et al. 1989; Sterns 1987; Weissman and Weissman 1989). Although psychiatric patients with polydipsia frequently have mild, chronic hyponatremia, a bout of water drinking can precipitously further lower the serum [Na+] and cause symptoms of water intoxication.

The physiology of hyponatremia has been well-studied in animals (Arieff et al. 1976; Sterns et al. 1989, 1991; Verbalis 1989; Verbalis and Gullans 1991; Verbalis and Martinez 1991). As water intoxication develops and the serum [Na+] drops, an osmotic gradient forms between the brain and plasma. Water, which can pass freely through the blood-brain barrier, is driven into the brain. Several mechanisms are then activated to prevent osmotic swelling of the brain. An immediate rise in hydrostatic pressure in the brain increases the flow of fluid from the interstitial spaces into the CSF (Berl 1990b; Verbalis 1989). Brain sodium concentration falls within 30 minutes, and brain potassium decreases over several hours (Sterns and Spital 1990; Verbalis 1989). Electrolyte loss is complete within 5–7 hours (Sterns et al. 1989), which diminishes the osmotic difference between brain and plasma. Whereas brain water content does rise in acute hyponatremia, the flow of fluid into the CSF and the loss of electrolytes limit the increase to less than half of what would have occurred without adaptation.

Initially, all volume regulation in hyponatremia is a result of fluid shifts and electrolyte loss. In chronic hyponatremia, however, only 69% of the observed volume regulation can be accounted for by these changes. Despite a 22%–27% drop in plasma and extracellular sodium, brain water increases by only 3%–6% (Verbalis and Gullans 1991). With sustained hyponatremia, brain water content declines to normal (Verbalis and Drutarosky 1988). Cationic loss during volume regulation is almost entirely caused by changes in sodium and potassium; however, only 44% of the observed decrease in anions can be attributed to chloride. Organic osmolytes account for the remainder of anionic loss (Thurston et al. 1987; Verbalis and Gullans 1991). The concentration of these intracellular, low molecular weight compounds slowly falls over 2 days after the development of hyponatremia, paralleling the return of brain water to normal. Organic osmolytes include polyols (myoinositol), methylamines (creatine), and amino acids (glutamic acid, glutamine, and taurine) (Sterns et al. 1991; Thurston et al. 1987; Verbalis and Gullans 1991). There may be other, as yet unidentified, substances either lost from cells or osmotically inactivated, which also contribute to volume regulation (Verbalis and Drutarosky 1988; Verbalis and Gullans 1991). Brain adaptation to hyponatremia is largely complete within 48 hours.

If hyponatremia is mild or develops gradually, the brain changes described above can easily compensate for the lowered osmolality of the serum and cerebral edema can be prevented. Significant brain swelling occurs if the rate of water influx and fall in serum [Na+] are more rapid than brain compensatory mechanisms. Animals and patients dying with acute hyponatremia may therefore have diffuse cerebral edema that, if severe, can cause brain herniation. Water intoxication does not cause focal, structural brain lesions (Helwig et al. 1935; Raskind 1974; Rowntree 1923).

Verbalis and Drutarosky (1988) studied the long-term cerebral effects of sustained hyponatremia in animals. Using continuous, subcutaneous infusion of a vasopressin analogue (1-deamino-[8-D-arginine] vasopressin) and a concentrated, nutritionally balanced diet, they were able to induce and maintain severe hyponatremia in rats. With their technique, the animals had neither significant weight loss nor renal escape from the antidiuresis. Only 2% of rats died within 3 weeks of the induction of hyponatremia. The surviving animals were clinically asymptomatic and exhibited normal behavior in feeding, movement, and grooming. No rat had seizures. After 21 days of severe hyponatremia (mean [Na+] was 112 mEq/L), brain water was normal. Brain sodium, potassium, chloride, and organic osmolyte concentrations were low, but not generally less than at 2 days after the development of hyponatremia.

In people, chronic hyponatremia usually develops with diuretic use or in the setting of chronic illness. Patients with congestive heart failure, Addison's disease, nephrotic syndrome, liver failure, or the syndrome of inappropriate secretion of antidiuretic hormone associated with disease or medication are prone to hyponatremia.

Whereas severe hyponatremia can be well tolerated if it evolves slowly, many patients are symptomatic. Patients with chronic hyponatremia have the same range of symptoms as those with acute hyponatremia, but symptoms are generally less severe. Thus, these patients may have an impaired sensorium, nausea, vomiting, malaise, anorexia, generalized weakness, dysarthria, gait disturbance, and muscle cramps (Daggett et al. 1982; Levinsky 1991; Sterns 1987). There may be personality change with irritability, confusion, or hostility. Seizures also can occur in chronic hyponatremia but are less common than in acute hyponatremia.

Chronic hyponatremia is not associated with structural brain damage. Patients dying with chronic hyponatremia usually show no pathological changes. Animals with severe, prolonged, uncorrected hyponatremia do not have structural brain lesions (Illowsky and Laureno 1987; Verbalis and Drutarosky 1988).

CENTRAL PONTINE AND EXTRAPONTINE MYELINOLYSIS

In 1959, Adams et al. described an unusual demyelinated lesion in the center of the basis pontis in four patients. Subsequent studies identified similar lesions in extrapontine areas as well as the pons (Gocht and Colmant 1987; J. E. Goldman and Horoupian 1981; Okeda et al. 1986; Wright et al. 1979). An association between myelinolysis and hyponatremia was first suspected in the 1970s (Tomlinson et al. 1976). Controlled studies in several animal species have now proven that myelinolysis can be caused by correction of hyponatremia, but myelinolysis is not seen in animals with sustained, untreated hyponatremia or in those with a rise in sodium from normal to hypernatremic levels (Illowsky and Laureno 1987; Kleinschmidt-Demasters and Norenberg 1981; Laureno 1983).

Myelinolysis is characterized pathologically by the focal loss of myelin. A decrease in the number of oligodendrocytes is accompanied by astrocytosis (Wright et al. 1979). In contrast to multiple sclerosis and other demyelinating diseases, the lesions lack an inflammatory response. Although neurons and axons may be affected in severe myelinolysis, they are usually remarkably preserved despite extensive myelin destruction. Symmetric extrapontine lesions are most common in the basal ganglia, thalamus, subcortical white matter, lateral geniculate body, and cerebellum (Gocht and Colmant 1987; J. E. Goldman and Horoupian 1981; Okeda et al. 1986; Wright et al. 1979).

Confusion and lethargy are often the first signs of neurological deterioration (Karp and Laureno 1993). Spastic quadriparesis resulting from corticospinal tract damage in the basis pontis is typical of myelinolysis (Adams et al. 1959). Pseudobulbar palsy from corticobulbar tract involvement causes dysarthria or mutism, dysphagia, and a brisk jaw jerk reflex. Other signs reflect myelinolytic lesions elsewhere in the brain. Pupillary and oculomotor abnormalities occur with midbrain involvement (Mani and Laureno 1986). Lesions affecting the basal ganglia produce movement disorders, such as parkinsonism, chorea, and dystonia (Dickoff et al. 1988; Grafton et al. 1988; Maraganore et al. 1992). Behavioral and cognitive changes reported in patients with myelinolysis include diminished comprehension, irritability, and personality change (Karp and Laureno 1993; Price and Mesulam 1987). Demyelination of the cerebellum or cerebellar peduncles causes ataxia (Steller et al. 1988).

Originally, it was only possible to diagnose myelinolysis pathologically. Current brain imaging techniques, magnetic resonance imaging (MRI) and computed tomography (CT) scanning, have enabled premortem diagnosis (DeWitt 1985; DeWitt et al. 1984; Gerard et al. 1987; G. M. Miller et al. 1988; Moriwaka et al. 1988; Rippe et al. 1987; Schroth 1984; P. D. Thompson et al. 1989). Myelinolytic lesions appear hypodense on CT scans. MRI is more sensitive than CT scan in detecting myelinolysis (Brunner et al. 1988, 1990; G.M. Miller et al. 1988; Moriwaka et al. 1988; Ragland et al. 1989; A.J. Thompson et al. 1988). On MRI, lesions are hyperintense on T2-weighted images (Figure 9–1) and hypointense on T1-weighted images (Figure 9–2). There is no edema or mass effect associated with myelinolytic lesions.

There is a lag between the onset of myelinolytic symptoms and the appearance of lesions on imaging studies. Scans obtained earlier than 2 weeks after the onset of neurological dysfunction may fail to show lesions (Gross and Bell 1982; Hazratji et al. 1983;

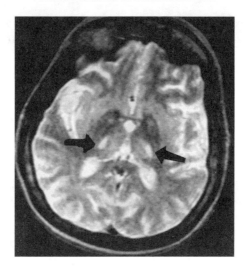

Figure 9–1. T2-weighted MRI image of extrapontine myelinolysis. Arrows indicate bilateral, symmetric myelinolytic lesions of the thalamus, which appear hyperintense.
Source. Reprinted from Laureno R: Neurologic syndromes accompanying electrolyte disorders, in *Handbook of Clinical Neurology*, Vol. 63. New York, Elsevier Science, 1993, pp. 545–573. Used with permission.

Rosenbloom et al. 1984). The absence of lesions on early imaging studies frequently makes the diagnosis of myelinolysis difficult.

In contrast to patients with uncorrected hyponatremia, those with myelinolysis have clearly localizing signs and symptoms, abnormal brain imaging studies, and pathological lesions. Other neurological evaluations also may be abnormal. In addition to generalized slowing, which may be difficult to differentiate from that seen in hyponatremic encephalopathy, the electroencephalogram in some patients with myelinolysis reveals focal slowing, low voltage, or burst-suppression pattern (Karp and Laureno 1993). CSF myelin basic protein levels are frequently elevated in patients with myelinolysis (Brunner et al. 1988; Kandt et al. 1983; Rosenbloom et al. 1984). Oligoclonal bands on CSF electrophoresis and high levels of CSF immunoglobulin G may also be present. Abnormal somatosensory, visual, and brainstem auditory evoked potentials

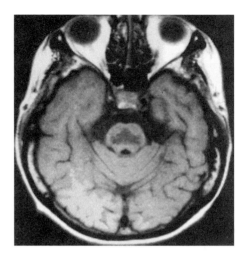

Figure 9–2. T1-weighted MRI image of central pontine myelinolysis. The large myelinolytic lesion appears hypointense and occupies the center of the basis pontis.
Source. Reprinted from Laureno R: Neurologic syndromes accompanying electrolyte disorders, in *Handbook of Clinical Neurology*, Vol. 63. New York, Elsevier Science, 1993, pp. 545–573. Used with permission.

have all been reported in myelinolysis (Brunner et al. 1988, Dickoff et al. 1988). Delayed conduction at the level of the brainstem on auditory evoked potentials may be especially useful in identifying a pontine lesion early in the course of myelinolytic illness when imaging studies are normal (Ingram et al. 1986).

Symptoms of myelinolysis do not immediately follow the rise in serum sodium, so that the overall course of illness in patients with myelinolysis is frequently biphasic. The initial symptoms are those of hyponatremic encephalopathy, which clear as the serum [Na+] rises. Deterioration as a result of myelinolysis begins 3–7 days later, at a time when the serum [Na+] is usually in the normal range.

Myelinolysis can be fatal; however, many patients survive. Maximal neurological dysfunction is reached about 1 week after correction of hyponatremia. Improvement in neurological function begins about 1 week later (i.e., 2 weeks after correction) and continues for up to 1 year in some patients (Karp and Laureno 1993). Some patients recover completely (Alberca et al. 1985; DeWitt et al. 1984; Kandt et al. 1983; Stam et al. 1984), whereas others have substantial residual disability (Clifford et al. 1989; Hazratji et al. 1983; Koci et al. 1990; D. S. Thompson et al. 1981). Persistent hemiplegia, spasticity, dysarthria, dysphagia, ataxia, and cognitive impairment may be disabling.

There is no treatment for myelinolysis. Steroids are not helpful, but medications are useful in treating specific symptoms such as parkinsonism or depression (Dickoff et al. 1988; Tinker et al. 1990). Physical therapy and good nursing care are essential to prevent contractures and infections in quadriplegic patients.

Myelinolysis can follow correction of hyponatremia of any cause. It may be more common in alcoholics, patients with liver disease, and debilitated patients (Adams et al. 1959; Estol et al. 1989; Wszolek et al. 1989) but has also been reported in otherwise healthy patients with hyponatremia caused by hyperemesis gravidarum, viral gastroenteritis, anorexia nervosa, bulimia, hypotonic fluid administration during surgery, and diuretic use (Brunner et al. 1990; Castillo et al. 1989; Copeland 1989; Estol et al. 1989; Greenberg et al. 1992; Wszolek et al. 1989).

PATHOPHYSIOLOGY OF CORRELATED HYPONATREMIA AND MYELINOLYSIS

Rapid correction of acute hyponatremia can return brain hydration to normal without adverse effects. However, a similar rise in serum sodium is dangerous if the brain has adapted to hyponatremia. As noted above, electrolyte and osmolyte levels fall to limit edema during a period of hyponatremia as short as 48 hours. When serum [Na+] rises during correction of hyponatremia, the brain becomes hypotonic relative to plasma and water is drawn from the brain. Sodium quickly reenters the brain extracellular fluid from the CSF. Replacement of intracellular potassium is not as rapid, occurring over several hours; repletion of organic osmolytes takes several days (Sterns et al. 1989; Verbalis and Gullans 1991b; Verbalis and Martinez 1991). Because electrolytes and osmolytes cannot be replaced quickly, patients with chronic hyponatremia are especially likely to develop significant brain dehydration if the serum [Na+] rises rapidly. Brain dehydration can be avoided by slow correction of chronic hyponatremia (Sterns et al. 1989).

Although myelinolysis has been reported following correction of acute hyponatremia (Brunner et al. 1990; Weissman and Weissman 1989), it is more likely to follow correction of chronic hyponatremia (Norenberg and Papendick 1984). It is especially likely if the serum [Na+] is allowed to reach hypernatremic levels during correction (Ayus et al. 1987). Although osmotic fluxes and brain dehydration may play a role in the development of myelinolysis, the pathogenetic mechanism of this disorder is not known. It has been hypothesized that areas of the brain affected by myelinolysis have in common an intermix of gray and white matter, which swell and contract differentially in response to osmotic changes, damaging myelinated fibers (Kleinschmidt-Demasters and Norenberg 1981, 1982; Messert et al. 1979). It has also been suggested that oligodendrocytes in perifascicular locations (as in the pons) are more prone to osmotic stress than those in interfascicular locations (Riggs and Schochet 1989).

The most critical factor for the development of myelinolysis is the rate of correction of hyponatremia. Retrospective analysis of human cases of myelinolysis and animal experimentation have shown that myelinolysis is more likely if the serum [Na+] rises quickly or undergoes a large increment within 48 hours (Arieff et al. 1992; Laureno 1983; Sterns et al. 1986; Verbalis and Gullans 1991; Verbalis and Martinez 1991). Based on these studies, it has been proposed that myelinolysis can be avoided if elevation of serum [Na+] is kept below 12 mEq/L in the first 24 hours of treatment or below 25 mEq/L in the first 48 hours of treatment (Arieff et al. 1992; Sterns et al. 1986). However, myelinolysis can occur in patients whose rise in serum [Na+] is within these guidelines (Gerber et al. 1983; Moriwaka et al. 1988; Price and Mesulam 1987). Myelinolysis has followed correction as gradual as 10 mEq/L in 24 hours and 21 mEq/L in 48 hours (Karp and Laureno 1993). An absolutely safe level of correction has not yet been established.

Hypertonic saline is commonly used to raise the serum sodium. Therefore, its use frequently precedes myelinolysis. Myelinolysis has also been reported following treatment with normal saline,

saline with furosemide, fluid restriction alone, oral sodium chloride, corticosteroids, and dialysis (Clifford et al. 1989; Grafton et al. 1988; Hazratji et al. 1983; Oh et al. 1989; Peces et al. 1988; Price and Mesulam 1987; Tanneau et al. 1988; Walker and Englander 1988; Zegers de Beyl et al. 1983).

MYELINOLYSIS IN POLYDIPSIC PATIENTS

Psychiatric patients with polydipsia frequently have a combination of acute and chronic hyponatremia. Mild chronic hyponatremia can be caused and maintained by the continuous ingestion of large quantities of fluids along with impaired free water excretion caused by the syndrome of inappropriate secretion of antidiuretic hormone or a reset osmostat. A drinking binge can suddenly drop the serum [Na+] and superimpose acute, symptomatic hyponatremia, which can be life-threatening. Polydipsic patients with acute hyponatremia treated with fluid restriction usually have a brisk diuresis and need no other specific measures to raise the serum sodium concentration. Some patients may require hypertonic saline.

Myelinolysis has been reported in polydipsic patients following correction of hyponatremia. Haibach et al. (1987) described a schizophrenic woman with self-induced vomiting and water drinking who became quadriplegic and mute 8 days after treatment of severe hyponatremia. Autopsy showed pontine myelinolysis. Silbert et al. (1992) reported a patient drinking 4–6 L of water per day for "cleansing." Behavioral changes, dysarthria, and ataxia developed 9 days after correction of hyponatremia. MRI revealed myelinolytic lesions in the pons and basal ganglia.

In contrast, Cheng et al. retrospectively evaluated the records of 13 polydipsic, psychiatric patients with hyponatremia-related seizures (1990). All patients survived rapid correction of hyponatremia. Myelinolysis was not detected (Gerber et al. 1983; Moriwaka et al. 1988; Price and Masulam 1987). Some cases of myelinolysis may have been missed because not all of the patients were followed closely and not all were scanned by MRI. Their study does, however, indicate that many polydipsic patients with acute, symptomatic hyponatremia tolerate rapid correction well.

Myelinolysis also can occur in psychiatric patients with hypo-natremia resulting from causes other than polydipsia such as di-uretic use, gastroenteritis, or burns (Cohen et al. 1991; Illowsky 1990; McColl and Kelly 1992). At times, behavioral changes as a result of myelinolysis may be difficult to differentiate from the patient's un-derlying psychiatric symptoms (McColl and Kelly 1992).

MANAGEMENT OF HYPONATREMIA

Myelinolysis is an uncommon illness. Most hyponatremic patients do not develop myelinolysis regardless of the speed of treatment (Sterns 1990). However, the possibility of iatrogenic myelinolysis exists and should be considered by physicians caring for hypo-natremic patients. A rational plan of management should attempt to minimize both morbidity from untreated hyponatremia and the risk of myelinolysis with its correction. Patients with acute hyponatremia differ from those with chronic hyponatremia in the severity of symptoms, in brain adaptation to hyponatremia, and in the risk of myelinolysis with correction. It is therefore impor-tant to determine the duration of hyponatremia before initiating treatment. In hospitalized patients, the onset of hyponatremia may be known. In outpatients, the duration of hyponatremia can only be estimated by noting the onset of symptoms or precipitating fac-tors, such as water drinking, diuretic use, or nausea and vomiting. When the duration is not clearly known, hyponatremia should be considered chronic.

Patients with acute hyponatremia are more likely to suffer sei-zures and die from water intoxication than those with chronic hyponatremia and are less prone to myelinolysis with a rise in se-rum sodium concentration. In acutely hyponatremic polydipsic pa-tients, fluid restriction alone may be all that is needed. Once fluid intake is controlled, many psychiatric patients with polydipsia have a rapid diuresis and return to normonatremia (Sterns 1990). In other severely symptomatic patients rapid correction requires saline administration. 3% saline can be used. Infusion at a rate of 1–2 ml/kg/hour raises the serum sodium concentration by 1–2 mEq/L/hour (Sterns 1990). Saline administration should be stopped and the rate of correction slowed once seizures are controlled or the patient's mental status improves. Hypertonic saline should be prepared in 100-ml bottles to avoid accidental overtreatment (Daggett et al. 1982). Electrolyte levels must be carefully monitored throughout the period of correction because the administration of hypertonic saline may combine with diuresis to raise the serum sodium concentration faster than expected. It has been proposed that cautious hypotonic fluid infusion can be used to prevent the serum sodium from rising too quickly in a patient who begins excreting large volumes of urine (Sterns 1990).

Whereas it cannot always be assumed that severely ill patients have acute hyponatremia, the absence of symptoms does suggest that hyponatremia is mild or chronic. Asymptomatic patients do not require aggressive correction. Treatment of an underlying illness such as the syndrome of inappropriate secretion of antidiuretic hormone or gastroenteritis, discontinuing diuretics, or removing precipitating factors may be all that is needed.

The risks of untreated hyponatremia and myelinolysis must be most carefully balanced in patients with symptomatic, chronic hyponatremia. Patients with impaired mentation or seizures require rapid correction. Saline infusion is commonly used in addition to treating the syndrome of inappropriate secretion of antidiuretic hormone or other underlying disease, discontinuing medications contributing to hyponatremia, and fluid restriction. Oral salt supplementation and corticosteroids are occasionally prescribed but are usually not necessary. Whereas hypertonic saline is frequently given, isotonic saline may adequately treat hyponatremia and allow more gradual correction. In hypovolemic patients, the use of half-normal saline may both provide volume expansion and avoid overcorrection (Oh et al. 1989). It has been suggested that the addition of furosemide or urea may lessen the risk of myelinolysis (Van Reeth and Decaux 1989). Regardless of the method of treatment, the increment in serum sodium should be kept below 10 mEq/L in the first 24 hours of treatment and below 21 mEq/L in the first 48 hours of treatment to the extent possible. The rate of correction should be slowed even further as soon as the patient is stable. Frequent blood sampling is crucial to determine the effect of saline administration on electrolyte levels and guide further treatment.

SUMMARY AND CONCLUSIONS

The brain's ability to adapt to hyponatremia can be overwhelmed by a large or sudden fall in plasma osmolality. Seizures, coma, and death from cerebral herniation can occur if acute hyponatremia is not treated. In contrast, adaptation to chronic hyponatremia is so complete that brain water content becomes normal despite sustained low plasma osmolality. Many patients with chronic hyponatremia are therefore able to tolerate extremely low serum sodium concentrations with few signs or symptoms. Rapid correction of hyponatremia once adaptation has occurred is not necessary and, in fact, may be dangerous because such patients are at particular risk of developing CNS myelinolysis from correction.

All hyponatremic patients, including psychiatric patients with polydipsia, should be treated as cautiously as possible. Patients whose symptoms are mild are best managed by removal or treatment of precipitating factors and restricted fluid intake. If the duration of hyponatremia is known to be brief and if seizures or a diminished level of consciousness are present, rapid correction may be life-saving. If hyponatremia has been present longer than the 48 hours required for cerebral adaptation or if the duration of hyponatremia is not known, gradual correction of the sodium deficit is warranted. Hypertonic saline infusion may be necessary. To the extent possible, the rise in serum sodium should be kept below 10 mEq/L in the first 24 hours of treatment and below 21 mEq/L in the first 48 hours of treatment.

Chapter 10

Management of Polydipsia and Hyponatremia

Robert A. Leadbetter, M.D., Michael S. Shutty, Jr., Ph.D., Jon R. Hammersberg, M.D., Patricia B. Higgens, L.C.S.W., M.S.W., and Diane Pavalonis, M.S.N., M.B.A.

Polydipsia and intermittent hyponatremia in chronically mentally ill patients can result in severe biopsychosocial impairment including an elevated death rate if not properly identified (Vieweg et al. 1985a). It is imperative that mental health care providers recognize the signs and the symptoms of this syndrome considering its impact on the health, functioning, and quality of life of the affected patient. This chapter is intended to assist the treatment team that is faced with these challenges and help minimize the complications of this syndrome.

Diagnosis of water dysregulation usually is either fortuitous or related to one of the medical sequelae of the problem. Issues in the identification of the patient at risk including a differential diagnosis and assessment of the severity of polydipsic behaviors are discussed. A monitoring program, relying on body weight and supplemented by behavioral and laboratory assessments, is described and interventions are proposed. Long-term care is dependent on the patient's ability to self-monitor as well as on community resources.

IDENTIFYING POLYDIPSIA AND HYPONATREMIA

Patients suffering from water dysregulation may be seen by mental health care providers in a variety of settings and at various points in their illnesses. Patients may have dramatic acute symptoms of hyponatremia, with one or more of the several medical sequelae, or with some of the more general characteristics or risk factors associated with the syndrome. Unfortunately, the diagnosis is frequently missed until a generalized seizure occurs (Jose et al. 1979; Vieweg et al. 1984). From a body-systems perspective, water intoxication usually affects the neurological or psychiatric and cardiovascular systems, whereas chronic sequelae frequently affect the urinary tract, skeletal, and gastrointestinal systems. The presence of polydipsia and hyponatremia require that the clinician perform a differential diagnosis, determine the severity of water dysregulation, and begin monitoring and interventions.

Water Intoxication

A sudden decrease in serum sodium presents the most severe risk to the patient with water dysregulation. Therefore, all mental health care providers should be familiar with the central nervous system and physical stigmata of hyponatremia. Physical signs of fluid overload are particularly useful, because changes in the patient's mental status can be confused with the primary psychiatric illness. In the most severe cases, however, a dramatic drop in serum sodium can cause central nervous system irritability and encephalopathy.

Physical signs of hyponatremia include edema of the extremities, abdominal distention, periorbital puffiness, nausea, and vomiting. An elevation in blood pressure and pulse may indicate volume overload. The older patient may be vulnerable to congestive heart failure. A coarse tremor, ataxia, myoclonus, hyperreflexia, and muscle irritability indicate frank central nervous system compromise. This compromise can progress into partial or grand mal seizures, frank encephalopathy, delirium, coma, and death.

Mental status changes observed in water intoxication are easily confused with the patient's primary psychiatric illness (Arieff 1984; Fleischhacker et al.1987; Webb and Gehi 1981). Psychomotor manifestations include restlessness and pacing. Affective changes may include elevated mood or euphoria, lability, irritability, and angry outbursts. Usually it is the change from baseline that is important (i.e., a patient who has a blunted affect may suddenly become more animated). Worsening of psychosis, particularly in the afternoon, may indicate hyponatremia. Cognitive changes across patients include deficits in complex information processing such as mental flexibility and verbal fluency (Shutty 1994), whereas individual patients may suffer from impaired attention span and other neuropsychological deficits. Judgment frequently deteriorates as the patient becomes more confused. It is important to remember that a patient's response to hyponatremia is idiosyncratic; for example, some patients become more disorganized and confused, whereas others become withdrawn and somnolent. Using specific psychiatric and neuropsychological testing can aid in identifying the patient's particular response to hyponatremia.

MEDICAL SEQUELAE

A number of chronic medical sequelae can endanger the patient's physical health. Increased urine volume can result in a hypotonic bladder, hydronephrosis, and renal dysfunction. Urinary incontinence, urinary tract infections, and chronic perineal irritation frequently occur. We have successfully treated several patients with large postvoid residuals utilizing serial catherizations, with documented decreases in bladder size and improvement in urinary and renal functioning.

Distention of the gastrointestinal tract caused by water loading can cause nausea, vomiting, and abdominal pain. Chronic malabsorption, diarrhea, and malnutrition are not uncommon. Also, some patients will skip meals to allow greater weight gain. This effect can be detected by daily monitoring; interventions to ensure an appropriate diet follow. Chronic hypocalcemia has been documented (Vieweg et al. 1986d), although it is unclear whether it is a result of polyuria or poor absorption. As a result, osteopenia and increased vulnerability to fractures has been reported (Delva et al. 1989).

Other Presentations

Behaviors associated with polydipsia might include frequent trips to the bathroom, consumption of nonpotable water sources, and increased smoking. Hoarding of salt, cigarette butts, and instant coffee may occur. An instant coffee "black market" among patients facilitates its abuse, and polydipsic patients are particularly prone to this problem.

Changes in appearance (compared to baseline) are evident as patients neglect their personal hygiene and become disheveled. Alternatively we have seen patients who have become more fastidious with their grooming, although they neglect key features. Similarly, some patients become more socially withdrawn and isolated, whereas others develop a circle of fellow water drinkers who facilitate each other's access to fluids through sharing of cups, bringing drinks to a patient on fluid restriction, and so on.

Progression to Hyponatremia

The progression from the onset of psychosis to polydipsia and hyponatremia follows a predictable course in schizophrenia (Vieweg et al. 1989f). As a rule, a relentless increase in water consumption is noted early in the illness. An early sign of polydipsia in these patients is a morning specific gravity of less than 1.003 (Vieweg et al. 1984d). On a day-to-day basis, however, changes in water consumption may go undetected and can be difficult to substantiate. Indeed, patients may go months, if not a year or more, between exacerbations. It is important, therefore, to remain vigilant and intervene rapidly if indicated. Identifying what environmental cues and other determinants are associated with polydipsia can be useful.

After 5 or more years of polydipsia, episodic hyponatremia may begin to occur, perhaps dependent on environmental variables (Bugle et al. 1992). Factors that can predate development of frank hyponatremia include nicotine and caffeine abuse, treatment with anticholinergic or certain psychotropic medications, and substance abuse. Patients who have concurrent diagnoses of schizophrenia and alcohol abuse are particularly prone to polydipsia and hyponatremia (Ripley et al. 1989). A history of these factors along with suspected polydipsia indicates the need for further evaluation to rule out hyponatremia.

Differential Diagnosis

In the differential diagnosis of hyponatremia, the physician must rule out other medical conditions and medication effects that can mimic water dysregulation (M. Goldman 1991; Illowsky and Kirch 1988). Carbamazepine therapy, commonly used in the seriously mentally ill, is a frequent cause of hyponatremia. Patients with hypothyroidism, Cushing's syndrome, diuretic therapy, syndrome of inappropriate antidiuretic hormone secretion (as a result of certain carcinomas or head injury), and nicotine use (Allon et al. 1990) also can be present with hyponatremia.

Polydipsia and polyuria may be caused by diabetes insipidus. Hypothalamic disorders, renal disorders, and medications, particularly lithium treatment, are the most common. It is particularly important to ensure that diabetes insipidus is not mistaken for polydipsia-hyponatremia, because fluid restriction is dangerous. Other notable causes of polydipsia include diabetes mellitus and anticholinergic medications. Syndromes associated with excessive antidiuretic hormone production have elevated urine osmolality (>100 mOsm), whereas in polydipsic-hyponatremic patients the urine usually is markedly dilute (< 100 mOsm).

ESTABLISHING THE SEVERITY OF POLYDIPSIA

Once a patient is suspected to have polydipsia and episodic hyponatremia, the degree of severity of water dysregulation should be established. Ideally, direct measurement of oral fluid intake would determine whether a patient is polydipsic. However, this method is impractical. Instead, a combination of approaches to assess drinking behavior may be used. Changes in the patient's body weight is the easiest method if done regularly in a standardized fashion as described in the following section. We also sample the patient's actual drinking behavior using a standardized behavioral observation scale. As a way of corroborating the information, "spot" urine creatinines can be used to estimate fluid consumption.

A behavior sampling method (Virginia Polydipsia Scale) has been developed to assess drinking behaviors. The scale has shown excellent interrater reliability and sensitivity to changes in psychiatric functioning caused by polydipsia (Shutty et al. 1992). Patients are unobtrusively observed using a standard protocol for several hours a day to determine idiosyncratic drinking patterns. The Virginia Polydipsia Scale involves observation of patient activities before and after any bout of drinking, the number of cigarettes consumed, urine volume, drinking source, rate of drinking, time drinking occurs, and amount drunk. In addition, the Virginia Polydipsia Scale measures 20 psychiatric symptoms (e.g., angry outbursts, social withdrawal, pacing) frequently associated with water intoxication.

In general, behavioral assessment has highlighted specific differences between polydipsic-hyponatremic patients and psychiatric control subjects. For example, polydipsic patients do not drink more frequently than matched control subjects but do drink greater volumes with each drinking bout. They do not void as much nor as often as control subjects. These findings are helpful clinically because they suggest that time spent at the water source drinking is more crucial than mere number of times drinking occurs. Specific behavioral interventions rely on this kind of information. In the individual case, behavioral sampling can help specify drinking risk periods, idiosyncratic patterns of drinking, and idiosyncratic responses to water loading. Whenever a specific behavioral management plan is indicated, behavior observations can be used to help design, implement, and evaluate subsequent behavioral interventions.

If use of behavior sampling is not possible, documenting polydipsia without hyponatremia may be done through laboratory evaluation. Abnormalities are consistent with water loading, diuresis, and inappropriate antidiuretic hormone secretion. Frequently, serum osmolality is decreased, yet urine osmolality indicates less than maximal dilution. Serum hypocalcemia resulting from diuresis may be noted. Urine specific gravities are frequently in the 1.000–1.005 range. Even more accurate are urine creatinines. Because creatinine is constantly excreted, one can estimate 24-hour urine volume by obtaining several urine creatinines at scheduled intervals throughout the day, averaging them, and using the formula:

Males: $\dfrac{20 \text{ mg/kg} \times \text{patient weight (kg)}}{\text{Mean urine creatinine (mg/dl)}} \times 0.1 \text{ (L/dl)} = \text{urine volume (in L)}$

Females: $\dfrac{15 \text{ mg/kg} \times \text{patient weight (kg)}}{\text{Mean urine creatinine (mg/dl)}} \times 0.1 \text{ (L/dl)} = \text{urine volume (in L)}$

MONITORING PROCEDURES

Once it has been established that a patient has severe polydipsia and intermittent hyponatremia, a reliable way of monitoring the patient's acute risk for hyponatremia should be implemented. Several studies promote using the patient's body weight as an indirect method to estimate fluid overload and therefore risk for hyponatremia (Delva and Crammer 1988; Godleski et al. 1989; M. B. Goldman and Luchins 1987; Vieweg et al. 1990c). For most patients, a water weight gain of 1 lb will reduce the serum sodium by one mEq/L. It is important to remember that using the body weight is not only a method of monitoring but is also an intervention.

Our group has developed a comprehensive monitoring procedure using a monthly weight chart. This chart employs a "base" weight and a daily weight allowance to intervene before severe hyponatremia occurs. This protocol allows for adjustment of the "base" weight, improves the prediction of actual low serum sodiums, and simplifies the estimation of the serum sodium throughout the day. The following is a detailed description of how to implement monitoring procedures.

Weight Chart

Figure 10–1 shows a typical monthly weight chart of a patient. Separate charts for each patient are kept in a notebook for easy analysis and revision. On this chart the daily morning (6 A.M.) weight is

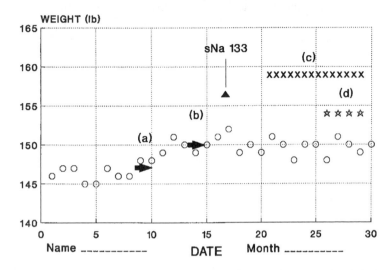

Figure 10–1. Weight chart: a) base weight, b) reset base weight, c) daily weight allowance, d) A.M. limit.

identified as a circle, and the afternoon (4 P.M.) weight as a triangle. Serum sodiums are noted adjacent to the weight at the time the sodium was drawn. Morning and afternoon weight limits are recorded on the weight chart, as discussed below.

Base Weight

The patient is weighed after arising in the morning and before beginning to consume fluids. After several daily measurements, it becomes clear that morning weights tend to oscillate around a "base weight," which is identified on the weight chart (Figure 10–1) with an arrowhead (a).

All subsequent monitoring depends on an accurate base weight. Minor fluctuations (a pound or two) in morning weight are expected and require no action. Temporary deviations of several pounds occur, for example, when the patient eats a salty pizza late in the evening (raising the weight) or after a bowel movement (lowering the weight) and do not require changes in the base weight.

However, when a change of several pounds persists for several days, it is necessary to "reset" the base weight (Figure 10–1b).

Daily Weight Allowance

Once the base weight is established, the 4 P.M. weight limit is determined. This limit is calculated by obtaining a 4 P.M. serum sodium concentration and correlating it with the 4 P.M. weight. Remembering the 1 mEq/lb relationship, the 4 P.M. serum sodium is used to predict the weight at which the serum sodium would fall to 130; that weight is identified as the patient's "P.M. limit" on the weight chart. The P.M. limit is marked with a line of X's (X-X-X). The difference between base weight and the 4 P.M. limit is the daily weight allowance (Figure 10–1c).

For example, Jim's usual morning weight is 150 lbs. His laboratory tests are done routinely at 6 A.M. and 4 P.M. on Wednesdays. Wednesday afternoon at 4 P.M. his weight was 156 lbs and his serum sodium was 133. The sodium will drop 1 mEq/lb of weight gain, and thus his sodium is predicted to fall to 130 at 159 lbs (156 + 3). The afternoon weight limit is set at 159 lbs. His daily weight allowance is 9 lbs.

Assuming a normal serum sodium associated with the base weight, 3–4 lbs of the daily allowance in the morning is allowed, identifying it as "A.M. limit." A line of stars (☆-☆-☆) is used to mark the A.M. limit on the weight chart (Figure 10–1d). By serially following the A.M. weight, patients who have begun drinking during the night can be detected. This prevents missing a patient who may already be in trouble.

Weight Table

Once the total daily allowance is known, incremental increases in weight allotment are distributed throughout the day between 6 A.M. and 4 P.M.. A weight table (Figure 10–2) is used, which the nursing staff can consult during the day. Patients who gain large amounts of weight quickly, or who are severely polydipsic on a regular basis, need to be weighed as often as hourly. More typically, patients get into trouble on a once-every-few-days to once-

Name_____

"Base Weight"

If _____ weight exceeds _____ pounds plus

6 A.M.	_____	_____
8 A.M.	_____	_____
10 A.M.	_____	_____
12 noon	_____	_____
2 P.M.	_____	_____
4 P.M.	_____	_____
6 P.M.	_____	_____
8 P.M.	_____	_____

              then   then

     Restrict to ward[1]   Obtain serum sodium
                                       immediately[2]

1. Until patient loses _____ pounds
2. On nights or weekends, nurse may elect to give po NaCl (per note 3)
3. 4.5 grams NaCl po for serum sodium $\leq$ 129 mEq/L;
   Repeat po NaCl in 2 hours if serum sodium is $\leq$ 126 mEq/L.
4. If 4 P.M. serum sodium is $\leq$ 126 mEq/L, then repeat serum sodium in A.M.

Figure 10–2. Weight table.

every-few-weeks basis; they need only to be weighed twice a day. Staff can choose to weigh as needed if polydipsia is suspected.

    The weight table is kept with the patient's weight chart. Every time the base weight is changed on the weight chart, it is also changed on the weight table. The hourly increments on the weight table are revised much less frequently and only when indicated by unexpected serum sodium levels.

Adjusting the Protocol

The daily weight allowance should be decreased if indicated serum sodiums are consistently < 130 or increased if serum sodiums are persistently normal at either A.M. or P.M. weight limits. New weight increments are written on the time lines appropriate for the patient (Figure 10–2). New limit lines are drawn on the weight chart (Figure 10–1).

For example, Jim's base weight is stable at 150 lbs, but his 4 P.M. weights are consistently at his limit of 159 lbs. Serum sodiums at 4 P.M. (159 lbs) have been 133. We are confident he has not been eating salt. His protocol can be "loosened" by raising his P.M. limit 3 lbs from 159 to 162 (where the serum sodium is now expected to be 130). Because his base weight is still 150 lbs, he can now gain 12 lbs during the day without restrictive intervention or getting blood drawn to measure serum sodium.

His weight table would look something like this:

If weight exceeds (150) plus...

6 A.M.	3	4 (arbitrarily start with 4)
8 A.M.	5	6 (breakfast allowance)
10 A.M.	6	7
12 noon	7	8
2 P.M.	9	10 (lunch allowance)
4 P.M.	11	12 (4 P.M. Target)
6 P.M.	12	13
8 P.M.	13	14

The serum sodium (rightmost) column is filled in first and then the "Restrict" column is completed by subtracting 1 lb. See Figure 10–2.

Accuracy in Weighing and Other Pitfalls

It is critical to follow a consistent technique in weighing to ensure reliability of monitoring. To weigh a patient accurately, all sweaters, coats, and shoes should be removed before the patient steps on the scales. The patients pockets should be emptied and the patient should be encouraged to void before being weighed. The patient should stand upright, with feet close together, in the middle of the scale platform with arms at the side.

Other problems include staffing patterns, staff knowledge, patient compliance, and monitoring during passes. Nursing staff levels may be increased during the morning weight collection. All staff are provided several weeks of training on the weight protocol and receive regular updates. We attempt to minimize restriction of the patient's rights unless his or her weight indicates a serum sodium level of < 130 mEq/L. If a patient refuses to cooperate with a weigh-in, we assume the patient is in trouble and intervene accordingly. When patients are going on day passes with family members, relatives are asked to discourage excessive fluid consumption. On overnight passes, the family is given weight parameters to follow and is educated about the signs and the symptoms of hyponatremia.

A problem with using the patient's body weight to predict hyponatremia is intermittent salt consumption. When trying to determine why patients were exceeding their daily weight allowance but had normal serum sodiums, we observed actual table salt hoarding. When interviewed, patients volunteered that they felt an urge to consume salt and thought it would help their "salt level." It is not clear whether this behavior was intended to alter the weight allowance or caused by an increased salt appetite associated with hyponatremia (Shutty et al. 1993).

INTERVENTIONS BASED ON WEIGHT GAIN AND TREATMENT OF ACUTE WATER INTOXICATION

The methods described above function as a treatment as well as a method of monitoring. The target weight protocol involves shaping of patient behavior where the primary goal is self-regulation of fluid consumption. Patients are rewarded with privileges for maintaining a low weight, and patients with increased water weight are restricted. In addition, the frequency of weighings (an event many patients perceive as bothersome) is reduced during periods of good weight control. Hence, control of weight is rewarded by decreased treatment intervention. Yet, it is important to intervene before the patient reaches the point where behavioral control becomes more difficult and more restrictive levels of intervention are required. Most importantly, patients identified as having acute hyponatremia need immediate treatment to prevent the complications previously outlined.

Serum Sodium Determinations

Routinely a STAT serum sodium is obtained any time the patient's weight exceeds the weight indicated on the weight table, which is estimated to correlate with a serum sodium < 130. A STAT serum sodium is also obtained any time the patient suddenly gains an unusual amount of weight. There are three reasons to determine STAT serum sodium levels when the patient is over the weight limit:

1. to evaluate the potential danger to the patient, because profound hyponatremia is life-threatening.
2. to assess the validity of the limit. Our approximation of a limit may be incorrect. The more data obtained, the more confidently the limit can be set. If a prediction of a serum sodium of 130 is made and it is actually 134, the afternoon weight limit might safely be raised (see exceptions below).
3. to guide intervention. If the serum sodium is ≤ 129, oral salt is usually given (see exceptions below.)

Brittle or Tolerant Patient

Some patients who weight 120 lbs can drink 12 lbs of water without dropping their sodium. Conversely, some patients who weigh 180 lbs can drop their sodium after an ingestion of 4 lbs of water. Until the individual's pattern is established, it is safer to obtain every "indicated" serum sodium level. When the patient's pattern becomes clear, night and weekend serum sodiums may be made optional. Refer to Figure 10–2.

Serum Sodium Levels

When a patient gains weight to within 1 lb of the limit for a given time of day (estimated serum sodium of 132–130 mEq/L), the patient is restricted to the ward and redirected from fluid sources. Refer to Figure 10–2.

When the serum sodium is ≤ 129, 4.5 grams of oral sodium chloride are given if there are no contraindications such as congestive heart failure or hypertension. The patient is directed to the bed area or a quiet room that can be directly observed from the nurse's station. Hourly weights are obtained until several pounds of water weight have been lost.

If the serum sodium is ≤ 126, 4.5 grams of salt are given and the dose is repeated in 2 hours. Otherwise the intervention is as above, except that a morning serum sodium is obtained the following day.

If the patient's serum sodium is < 124 or has dropped rapidly, absolute water restriction, seizure precautions, and direct continuous observation are implemented. If the patient is extremely hyponatremic (serum sodium < 120 mEq/L) or if changes in level of consciousness or obtundation occur, then immediate transfer to an appropriate medical setting for treatment is initiated. Intravenous correction of severe hyponatremia should be done cautiously because of the risk of central pontine myelinolysis.

EXTENDED CARE

Immediate interventions, as outlined above, do not address the long-term management of patients with polydipsia and intermittent hyponatremia. Unfortunately many patients are not able to decrease fluid consumption sufficiently to prevent episodes of hyponatremia. A longer-term management perspective needs to be taken to improve the patient's quality of life and decrease the need for restrictive and staff-intensive interventions.

Extended care interventions are broken down into psychosocial, behavioral, and medical domains. Patient awareness and self-monitoring of fluid consumption and weight changes can be translated into community living settings. Psychosocial interventions support this approach by changing enduring patterns of behavior. When necessary, individualized behavioral programs can be developed for those who fail broader interventions. Finally, a number of medications have been proposed for the prophylactic treatment of hyponatremia, although further studies are needed.

Psychosocial Interventions

Successful long-term care depends on the patient's own ability to limit polydipsia. One way to assess this ability is to examine the patient's subjective reasons for polydipsia. Many patients note a euphoric quality associated with polydipsia, although others admit to increased irritability. Some explain polydipsia based on delusional ("to wash out the demons") or health reasons ("my doctor told me to drink eight glasses of water a day"), yet most patients note a desire for stimulation, similar to other substances of abuse. Developing an understanding of what drives polydipsia can improve management.

In association with these assessments, we have instituted a "Water Drinker's Group" to aid a patient's self-control. When a patient first arrives on the ward, introduction to the group helps patients identify polydipsia as a health problem and encourages them to talk freely about their drinking patterns and efforts to reduce drinking. Recognition that fellow patients also suffer from the syndrome aids in breaking down denial and begins the process of rehabilitation. Patients can become readily engaged in talking about their polydipsia over a brief period (approximately 4–6 weeks) and can learn basic facts about the syndrome and its complications. Group topics typically include repeated progress checks on patients' ability to self-monitor and control their drinking during the past week, education about hyponatremic states, and the development of strategies to reduce drinking. Finally, group therapy provides corrective feedback and encouragement to those patients who are involved in intensive behavioral protocols.

Interventions throughout the ward that discourage fluid consumption include confiscation of drinking cups and cans, monitoring bathroom privileges, redirection from the water fountain, and regulating coffee and soda intake. The frequency and severity of water intoxication determines the level of privileges a patient earns. These privileges include time off the ward, time off hospital grounds, ability to participate in rewarding activities, and so on. These interventions take place on an open unit and minimize dependence on artificial structure. As a result, they are generalizable to other settings such as community residential treatment programs.

Behavioral Interventions

For patients who have failed to respond to interventions and group therapy, more intensive behavioral interventions for specific patients are developed. Individual treatment plans are used whenever a particular patient is poorly managed by the ward milieu alone. Behavioral interventions have been reported to be successful in reducing fluid intake (Klonoff and Moore 1984; McNally et al. 1988). These studies depended on regulating all sources of fluid, which can be difficult. Others have suggested a token economy or point system that is connected to compliance with weight parameters.

We successfully treated an otherwise refractory patient with polydipsia and intermittent hyponatremia using an individualized behavioral treatment program without regulating all fluid sources (Pavalonis et al. 1992). A reinforcement schedule contingent on weight gain secondary to water intake was employed. This intervention resulted in a decrease in estimated fluid consumption from 10 to 4 L per day, which persisted at 1 year follow-up. Incidents of hyponatremia decreased by 62%.

Medication Interventions

Acute antipsychotic and anxiolytic treatment can reduce the impulsive, psychotic, and anxiety-driven nature of water consumption. Long-term success, however, depends on trying to prevent hyponatremia. Lithium, which blocks the effect of antidiuretic hormone on the renal tubules increasing free water excretion, can lessen the severity of hyponatremic episodes (Vieweg et al. 1988k). However, lithium can enhance arginine vasopressin (AVP) release (Gold et al. 1983b), and the clinical effectiveness of this treatment needs verification (Alexander et al. 1991; A. T. Riggs et al. 1991). Phenytoin may decrease AVP release (Fichman et al. 1970) as well as prevent seizures. Demeclocycline, which also blocks AVP's effect on the kidneys, has been used with some success (Goldman and Luchins 1985; Nixon et al. 1982; Vieweg et al. 1988k), although recent studies have questioned the efficacy of this treatment (Alexander et al. 1991).

Our group recently has found that clozapine treatment can be effective in patients with polydipsia and hyponatremia. In contrast to standard antipsychotic treatment, there was a significant improvement in hyponatremia and an apparent decrease in fluid consumption. Across eight patients, the average routine 4 P.M. serum sodium was 133.6 mEq/L pre-clozapine and 136.6 mEq/L post-clozapine (t (7) = $-$ 4.42, $P < 0.003$). The average number of days out of 26 weeks that patients gained more than 5% of their baseline (6 A.M.) body weight was 32.2 days pre-clozapine and 5.4 days post-clozapine, approaching statistical significance at ($t(7) = 2.23, P < 0.06$). The average amount of fluid drunk as calculated from diurnal urine creatinines was 6.67 L pre-clozapine and 4.66 L post-clozapine, approaching statistical significance at $t(5) = 2.10, P < 0.09$. Although clozapine treatment looks very promising, these results need to be replicated.

COMMUNITY CARE

Patients with a serious mental illness ordinarily require extensive discharge planning and community case management. The combination of a severe mental illness and polydipsia-hyponatremia syndrome requires the development of intensive and well-coordinated discharge plans. Most mental health providers, family members, and patients themselves are not aware of the danger of polydipsia and hyponatremia and its sequelae.

Before discharge a patient should be assessed for ability to monitor and self-regulate fluid intake. It is important to examine the patient's level of insight and acceptance, motivation, and cognitive skills. Those patients with deficits in these areas can be referred to supervised living situations where some form of external structure and monitoring is available. In planning any transition to community living, a series of passes is attempted before discharge. During the pass, the patient records his or her body weight and is instructed how to handle elevated weights. The frequency and severity of weight gain while on a pass reflects the patient's readiness for discharge and indicates the level of structure needed.

Education

Education of the patient, family members, and community care providers is fundamental to successful discharge. Typically, each patient has an individualized weight protocol to track diurnal weights and estimated sodium levels. The purpose and the importance of these plans is emphasized to the patient's community care providers. Educational objectives include familiarizing aftercare providers with the patient's particular hyponatremic symptom constellation. This procedure eliminates unnecessary changes in antipsychotic medications after discharge and improves the competence of community care providers.

We have had particular difficulty when discharging patients on either salt regimens for excessive weight gain or the use of phenytoin. Physicians unfamiliar with these treatments are reluctant to continue them without traditional indications. It is important that this information be outlined for community based providers.

Resource Availability

Considering the obvious limitations in obtaining immediate medical attention in the community, it is important that discharge planning assess the resources that are available to the patient. If family members, significant others, or mental health staff are available to aid the patient with monitoring, then the discharge process is much simpler. Fortunately weight scales are cheap and readily available; they are a necessary part of the discharge of intermittently hyponatremic patients. It is worthwhile to have a laboratory, or emergency department facility, available in cases where the serum sodium is thought to be dangerously low.

CONCLUSION

Polydipsia and intermittent hyponatremia can present the clinician with challenging management problems. Successful treatment is contingent on the cooperativeness of the patient and a well-organized treatment strategy. The clinician faces challenges with identification, monitoring, interventions, long-term care, and discharge planning. A well-coordinated approach can minimize the impact of water dysregulation on the patient's health, psychosocial functioning, and quality of life.

Chapter 11

Pharmacological Approaches to Disturbances in Water Regulation in Severely Mentally Ill Patients

William B. Lawson, M.D., Ph.D.

A s noted in previous chapters, severely mentally ill patients are at risk for developing polydipsia. That is, they drink fluids excessively, sometimes exceeding 10 L per day (Lawson et al. 1985). Frequently polydipsia is associated with releasing inappropriate arginine vasopressin, leading to the development of a dilutional hyponatremia, as free water excretion is inhibited (M.B. Goldman et al. 1988). Often no known causes can be identified (M. Goldman 1991). Both polydipsia and hyponatremia can lead to significant morbidity and mortality, accounting for as many as 18% of nongeriatric deaths in schizophrenic patients (Vieweg et al. 1985c).

Various techniques of water restriction, behavioral interventions, and even group therapy can be effective (M. B. Goldman and Luchins 1987; Millson et al. 1993) and are described elsewhere in this book. In most instances these techniques were used in structured inpatient settings. It is not clear whether these techniques would be as effective in less restrictive environments, a crucial issue in this era of deinstitutionalization. Moreover polydipsia with hyponatremia has been associated with patients who have severe psychopathology or cognitive impairment (Kirch et al. 1985; Lawson et al. 1985). These patients often lack the capacity to be cooperative with such approaches. Finally, disturbed water regulation is often a chronic condition, which further limits the effectiveness of pharmacological approaches. Pharmacological interventions would appear to be warranted in these severely impaired chronic patients. However, our review will show that proven clinical pharmacological options are limited.

ANIMAL MODELS

Part of the reason for the absence of pharmacological options may be the absence of adequate animal models. Substantial work has been done in the past decade to understand the physiology and the pharmacology of drinking behavior and water regulation in animal models that have emphasized mesolimbic dopaminergic pathways (see Chapters 3 and 5). Various animal models of schizophrenia also have put an emphasis on alterations in dopaminergic mesolimbic pathways (Lyons 1991). These pathways have also been implicated in drinking behavior both through lesion research and pharmacological probes (Dourish 1983). Unfortunately drinking behavior and water regulation have not been investigated in most presumptive animal models of schizophrenia.

Luchins (1990) has proposed, however, that rats with certain hippocampal lesions may be useful models for both schizophrenia and drinking disturbances, because hippocampal pathology has been implicated in schizophrenia and rats with such behavior may become polydipsic. Moreover, we recently developed an animal model for schizophrenia in which rats were given prenatal injections of amphetamine (Lyon et al. 1993). Preliminary results indicated that these rats developed polydipsia and a preference for alcohol. Alcoholism is common in schizophrenia and especially in patients who are polydipsic (Ripley et al. 1989). If confirmed, this finding will be one of the few instances in which a remote biochemical or structural intervention increased fluid intake or alcohol preference. Thus far, pharmacological interventions have not been used in either of the models described above to investigate ways of blocking polydipsia. Additional research with animal models could be useful in generating possible pharmacological interventions for clinical use.

SALT SUPPLEMENTATION

Supplementation with sodium salts is commonly used as an initial intervention in patients with hyponatremia. Supplementation has been carried out in two ways: by acute infusion or by chronic oral administration. Acute correction of the low serum sodium has been used to manage the hyponatremic seizures often seen in these patients or in the occasional patient with coma. However, rapid correction has been controversial because it may lead to central pontine myelinolysis, which can be associated with bulbar palsy, quadriplegia, coma, and death (Illowsky and Laureno 1987; Laureno and Karp 1988). Central pontine myelinolysis is extremely rare and the risks must be balanced against the risk of permanent structural damage or death. Nevertheless the clinician should be cautious because anticonvulsants can treat the seizures, patients seldom lose consciousness for more than a few minutes, and many patients will have a large spontaneous diuresis leading to self-correction of serum electrolytes (M. Goldman 1991). Generally, hypertonic saline can be considered when the patient does not rapidly regain consciousness and does not have cardiac, hepatic, or renal failure. Serum sodium can then be administered at a rate of 1–1.5 mEq/L per hour to a total increase of 12–15 mEq/L during the first 24 hours (Goldman 1991; Narins 1986).

Chronic use of salt tablets or Gatorade is safer and may have a role in preventing hyponatremic seizures. Vieweg et al. (1985e) reported some short-term efficacy in raising serum sodium and in preventing seizures in four patients. However the salt was rapidly lost in the urine, and progressively higher doses of salt were required to maintain normal serum sodium levels. In addition significant hypertension developed in two patients. De La Rocha et al. (1989) studied the effects of 4 grams/day of oral sodium on 14 psychiatric patients with hyponatremia over 16 weeks. Serum sodium, urine specific gravity, or body weight were not significantly affected. Blood pressure showed a statistically significant but clinically trivial elevation. A ward milieu program of drinking supervision was far more effective. We can therefore conclude that maintenance with oral sodium supplements offers little or no benefit for hyponatremic patients and has no advantage over behavioral techniques or various methods of fluid restriction (however, see Chapter 1 for a description of the use of salt tablets in the treatment of acute hyponatremia).

INHIBITION OF ANTIDIURETIC HORMONE

As noted above, psychiatric patients who develop hyponatremia appear to have inappropriate release of arginine vasopressin. Consequently agents that inhibit arginine vasopressin or its action at the kidney have been proposed as treatments. Lithium is known to produce a nephrogenic diabetes insipidus. It also has the advantage of being familiar to psychiatrists. It has been shown to be effective in open trials in some psychiatric patients with hyponatremia (Vieweg et al. 1985e, 1988k). Phenytoin also has transient vasopressin antagonist properties and has been shown to be effective in some psychiatric patients with hyponatremia when used in combination with lithium (Vieweg et al. 1988k). Although these agents can be effective, particularly when used in combination, significant problems have been associated with their use. First, these agents are not consistently effective (Decaux et al. 1989; Forrest et al. 1978; Kathol et al. 1986). Also, lithium directly stimulates thirst, has a low therapeutic index, and can become toxic at plasma levels close to therapeutic levels (De Soto et al. 1985; Nixon 1982).

The tetracycline demeclocycline is reportedly more effective in treating the syndrome of inappropriate antidiuretic hormone (SIADH) in nonpsychiatric patients and less toxic than lithium (Forrest et al. 1978). In psychiatric patients, demeclocycline has been found to be consistently effective in reducing the number of hyponatremic episodes and perhaps in reducing polydipsia in a double-blind controlled case report, an open case report, and two open clinical trials (M. B. Goldman and Luchins 1985; Khamnei 1984; Nixon et al. 1982; Vieweg et al. 1988l). A carefully done double-blind controlled study and a case report, however, did not find significant benefit (Alexander et al. 1991; Kathol et al. 1986).

Presumably, demeclocycline is not as consistently effective as the initial studies indicated. It also is expensive, promotes development of resistance to antibiotics, and has been associated with hepatic and renal toxicity (M. Goldman 1991). Moreover, vasopressin antagonists generally do not affect fluid intake. The medical consequences of a persisting polydipsia would still be present. Nevertheless these agents can provide benefit for some psychiatric patients at risk for developing significant hyponatremia and seizures.

ANTIPSYCHOTICS

Neuroleptics have been implicated as a cause of disturbed water regulation in psychiatric patients (Sandifer 1983). The anticholinergic effects of low-potency antipsychotics or the adjunctive anticholinergic agents frequently required by use of high-potency antipsychotics were believed to contribute to excessive fluid intake by inducing a dry mouth. Moreover, antipsychotics might cause or exacerbate hyponatremia by directly stimulating vasopressin release. The evidence that a dry mouth can cause polydipsia is surprisingly slim. Studies involving animal models and a review of the clinical literature indicated that restricted salivary flow will lead to polydipsia only with sapid solutions or as a response to the mechanical difficulty of eating, if at all (Lawson et al. 1974; Vance 1965). Although there are some undeniable case reports of antipsychotics causing SIADH, Sandifer (1983) noted that most of these reports did not involve rechallenges and half of the reports involved drug administrations of < 1 week. The incidence of antipsychotics producing SIADH is probably a rare phenomenon (Illowsky and Kirch 1988). Moreover, antipsychotics clearly are not the primary cause of most cases of polydipsia with or without hyponatremia because these disturbances in water regulation predated the neuroleptic era and were seen in medication-free patients (Illowsky and Kirch l988; Lawson et al. l985).

Animal studies rather consistently showed that dopamine blockers inhibited drinking behavior (Dourish 1983). Several reports indicated that both polydipsia and hyponatremia improved with antipsychotic therapy as psychosis improved (Hariprasad et al. 1980; Zubenko 1984). Interestingly, one case report indicated that the atypical antipsychotic molindone did not produce polydipsia and hyponatremia, but these disturbances were seen in the same patient with typical antipsychotics (Glusac et al. 1990).

The story with the atypical antipsychotic clozapine is clearer. A double-blind controlled case report by H. S. Lee et al. (1991) showed that unlike standard neuroleptics, clozapine was effective in reversing the diurnal variation in urine output noted to be a hallmark of the polydipsia seen in patients with disturbed water regulation. A subsequent open trial with multiple patients found a decrease in polydipsia and hyponatremia (Leadbetter et al. 1993). There is one report of clozapine causing hyponatremia (Ogilvie and Croy 1992). However, it is important to note that a rechallenge was not done, and idiopathic hyponatremia in a psychiatric patient cannot be excluded.

The rather consistent findings with clozapine strongly support the need for additional research. The mechanism is not easy to discern. Clozapine has greater efficacy than other antipsychotics (Kane et al. 1988). Clozapine's effectiveness in treating disturbed water regulation may be related to its overall greater efficacy in treating psychosis. On the other hand, clozapine's effectiveness may be related to its atypical features. Clozapine is a relatively weak dopamine D_2 blocker and does not cause the dramatic increase in prolactin seen with standard neuroleptics. Prolactin has an osmoregulatory role in lower species and may have a related role in humans that may involve increased risk for hyponatremia (Verghese et al. 1992). Clozapine has potent serotonergic, anticholinergic, and histaminergic activity (Baldessarini and Frankenburg 1991). Because many of these neurochemical systems are reported to be involved in water regulation in animal models, additional research is needed to clarify clozapine's mechanism of action (H. S. Lee et al. 1991).

Although clozapine appears to be a promising treatment, its side-effect profile limits its use. It has a significantly greater risk of causing agranulocytosis, which has led to a requirement of weekly white blood counts and restriction of its use to patients who do not respond to standard neuroleptics (Alvir et al. 1993). Moreover, a history of seizures are a relative contraindication because seizures are seen at higher doses (Baldessarini and Frankenburg 1991). Consequently, patients for whom the treatment would otherwise be appropriate might be excluded because of a history of hyponatremic seizures.

RENIN SYSTEM

Animal research has consistently implicated the renin-angiotensin system in drinking behavior. Angiotensin-II is one of the most potent dipsogens known and when injected intracerebrally will cause rats to drink themselves to death (Epstein 1987). This system probably has a limited role in the day-to-day regulation of thirst in humans, coming into play with substantial volume loss as in significant injury with loss of blood. Nevertheless it may be a factor in pathological drinking behavior. Captopril, an angiotensin-converting enzyme inhibitor, reversed polydipsia and hyponatremia in several case reports (J. A. Goldstein 1981, 1986; Vieweg et al. 1985d). We replicated the findings of Vieweg et al. of improved water metabolism and noted an improvement in mental status as well as water regulation in a single case (Lawson et al. 1988). We then conducted an open trial with six patients and found no benefit whatsoever. Another case study found no benefit, and one report suggested that captopril caused a fatal hyponatremic episode (Al-Mufti and Arieff 1985; Kathol et al. 1986). A more recent case report found enalapril, another angiotensin-converting enzyme inhibitor, to be effective in managing hyponatremia when captopril had no benefit (Sebastian and Bernardin 1990). Because enalapril is believed to be more centrally active, future research may focus on the more centrally active angiotensin-converting enzyme inhibitors.

Other Pharmacological Interventions

High-dose propranolol, a β-receptor blocker, was used to successfully treat a patient, based on the rationale that it may have some general benefit in schizophrenia and the finding that isoproterenol, a β-agonist, may increase thirst (Shevitz et al. 1980). Another case report found propranolol ineffective (Kathol et al. 1986). There have been no recent reports, suggesting that this treatment has been neglected or that others found no benefit and simply did not report it. Our experience is consistent with the latter interpretation. In an open trial using a similar methodology as with captopril, we found no benefit with doses of up to a gram per day. Because of the potential side effects and the low likelihood of success, pro- pranolol is not recommended for clinical use, although we did not find any significant adverse effects with a slow increase in dosage in otherwise healthy patients. Additional research may be feasible with the increasing availability of β-blockers with more specific action.

Primary polydipsia is often grouped with compulsive behavior, which led several investigators to give trials of fluoxetine, a specific serotonergic reuptake inhibitor currently approved for depression and recently approved for obsessive-compulsive disorder. M. B. Goldman and Janecek (1991) carefully studied five patients with a history of polydipsia and water intoxication and no other obses- sive-compulsive symptoms in an open trial. No consistent improve- ment was noted in a variety of indices. However, fluoxetine was effective in treating water intoxication in a patient with bulimia and other compulsive symptoms in addition to schizophrenia (Deas- Nesmith and Brewerton 1992). This case report is of interest because it suggests that fluoxetine may be effective in a subgroup of poly- dipsic patients with syndromes that are fluoxetine responsive. It cannot be determined from the case report whether bulimia or ob- sessive-compulsive variant was the underlying disorder.

Finally, given the extensive animal literature showing that opi- ate antagonists suppress fluid intake, Nishikawa et al. (1992) re- ported success with naltrexone, a long-acting opiate antagonist that can be taken by mouth, in a schizophrenic patient with water in- toxication. Vieweg and others (1985c) have proposed that these patients drink excessively because of the involvement of the opioid system, suggesting a "water addiction." Moreover the opiate an- tagonists are extremely safe. Additional research is warranted with these agents.

CONCLUSION

The literature is consistent in providing little in the way of guid- ance for the clinician because of the absence of a mechanism for the pathological condition, lack of studies in general, preponder- ance of case reports, and virtual absence of controlled trials. With the notable exception of the clozapine study, on methodological grounds alone virtually every study that showed efficacy can be criticized. Investigator bias and placebo effects often cannot be ruled out. The sizes of the samples were frequently inadequate. Moreover the condition spontaneously remits, making the interpretation of positive results difficult. In addition, the wide range of pharmacological interventions proposed thus far would suggest that some of these results are probably placebo responses. On the other hand, the paucity of studies also reflect the difficulties of doing research with this population of patients. These individuals often reside in settings where fiscal and administrative complexities impede the conduct of systematic investigations. Additional research in this field is clearly needed, especially trials consisting of double-blind, multisite studies.

The findings with clozapine certainly justify more research if only to have a new indication considered. In addition, there are now a number of new atypical antipsychotics undergoing study or recently approved. They tend to have more specificity of action then clozapine. If the efficacy of clozapine in treating water intoxication continues to be substantiated, a trial of the newer atypical agents is warranted for clinical reasons and to clarify the neurochemical system involved.

None of the findings with available agents contradict the caveat that after a workup and medication adjustments to rule out known causes of disturbed water regulation, various approaches to restrict fluid intake should be tried. If fluid restriction is not an option or is not workable in the long term, given the data that are available, the most reliable results have been found with various agents that address the hyponatremia. In the emergency situation, an argument can be made for saline infusion under the conditions described above to prevent central pontine myelinosis, although anticonvulsants also can be considered if the emergency is hyponatremic seizures. Phenytoin has the advantage of transiently treating the hyponatremia as well. For chronic care, agents such as demeclocycline or lithium/phenytoin combinations can be considered, keeping in mind that efficacy is not consistent. If possible, switching to an atypical antipsychotic should be considered. A trial of clozapine is certainly warranted if the patient qualifies under current Food and Drug Administration guidelines. If the patient has a seizure history, a review to exclude causes other than hyponatremia will be necessary. An angiotensin-converting enzyme inhibitor can also be considered, given the number of promising case reports. Other unproven agents that are relatively safe include selective serotonin reuptake inhibitors, antidepressants, and naltrexone. Above all, treatment of this disorder now remains an art that still requires the skillful hand of the flexible and innovative clinician.

References

Achard C, Ramond L: Potomanie chez un enfant. Bull Mem Soc Med Hop Paris 12:380–390, 1905

Ackerman U, Irizawa TG: Synthesis and renal activity of rat atrial granules depend on extracellular volume. Am J Physiol 247:R750–R752, 1984

Adams R, Victor M, Mancall EL: Central pontine myelinolysis: a hitherto undescribed disease occurring in alcoholic and malnourished patients. Arch Neurol Psychiatry 81:154–172, 1959

Adler RA, Herzberg VL, Brinck-Johnsen T, Sokol HW: Increased water excretion in hyperprolactinemic rats. Endocrinology 118:1519–1524, 1986

Adler S, Simplaceanu V: Effect of acute hyponatremia on rat brain pH and rat brain buffering. Am J Physiol 256:F113–F119, 1989

Adolph EF: Physiological Regulations. Lancaster, PA, Jacques Cattell Press, 1943

Adolph EF: Thirst and its inhibition in the stomach. Am J Physiol 161: 347–386, 1950

Adoph EF: Regulation of body water though water ingestions, in Thirst: Proceedings of the First International Symposium on Thirst in the Regulation of Body Water. Edited by Wayner MJ. Oxford UK, Pergamon, 1964, pp 5–14

Aiken JW, Vane RJ: Intrarenal prostaglandin release attenuates the vasoconstrictor activity of angiotensin. J Pharmacol Exp Ther 184:678–687, 1973

Ajlouni K, Kern MW, Tures JF, et al: Thiothixene induced hyponatremia. Arch Intern Med 134:1103–1105, 1974

Al-Mufti HI, Arieff AI: Captopril-induced hyponatremia with irreversible neurologic damage. Am J Med 79:769–771, 1985

Alberca R, Iriarte LM, Rasero P, et al: Brachial displegia in central pontine myelinolysis. J Neurology 231:345–346, 1985

Alexander RC, Illowsky-Karp B, Thompson S, et al: A double blind, placebo-controlled trial of demeclocycline treatment of polydipsia-hyponatremia in chronically psychotic patients. Biol Psychiatry 30:417–420, 1991

Alheid G, McDermott LJ, Kelly J, et al: Deficits in food and water intake after knife cuts that deplete striatal DA or hypothalamic NE. Pharmacol Biochem Behav 6:273–287, 1977

Allon M, Allen H, Deck L, et al: Role of cigarette use in hyponatremia in schizophrenic patients. Am J Psychiatry 147:1075–1077, 1990

Altshuler LL, Casanova MF, Sachdev N, et al: Shape and area of the hippocampus/parahippocampus in schizophrenic, suicide and control brains. Arch Gen Psychiatry 47:1029–1034, 1990

Alvir JM, Lieberman JA, Safferman AZ, et al: Clozapine induced agranulocytosis. N Engl J Med 3297:162–167, 1993

Alzheimer A: Beitrage zur pathologischen anatomie der hirnrinde und zur anatgomischen grundlage der psychosen. Mschr Psychiat Neurol 2:82–120, 1897

Anand BK, Brobeck JR: Hypothalamic control of food intake in rats and cats. Yale J Biol Med 24:123–140, 1951

Anderson B, Leksell LG, Lishajko F: Perturbations in fluid balance induced by medially placed forebrain lesions. Brain Res 99:261–275, 1975

Anderson RJ, Chung HM, Kluge R, et al: Hyponatremia: a prospective analysis of its epidemiology and the pathogenetic role of vasopressin. Ann Intern Med 102:164–168, 1985

Andersson B: Regulation of water intake. Physiol Rev 58:582–603, 1978

Andersson B, Rundgren M: Thirst and its disorders. Annu Rev Med 33: 231–239, 1982

Andersson B, Wyrwicka W: Elicitation of a drinking motor conditioned reaction by electrical stimulation of the hypothalamic "drinking area" in the goat. Acta Physiol Scand 41:194–198, 1957

Andreasen N, Nasrallah HA, Dunn V, et al: Structural abnormalities in the frontal system in schizophrenia: a magnetic resonance imaging study. Arch Gen Psychiatry 43:136–144, 1986

Andreasen NC: Negative symptoms in schizophrenia. Arch Gen Psychiatry 39:784–788, 1982

Andreasen NC, Ehrhardt JC, Swayze VW, et al: Magnetic resonance imaging of the brain in schizophrenia: the pathophysiological significance of structural abnormalities. Arch Gen Psychiatry 47:35–44, 1990

Andrews KM: Knife Cuts Through the Ventral Posterior Hypothalamus: Effects on Water Intake and Renal Functions. PhD dissertation, University of Chicago, 1993

Andrews KM, McGowan MK, Gallitano A, et al: Water intake during chronic preoptic infusions of osmotically-active or -inert solutions. Physiol Behav 52:241–246, 1992

Arieff AI: Central nervous system manifestations of disordered sodium metabolism. Endocrinol Metab Clin North Am 13:269–294, 1984

Arieff AI: Hyponatremia, convulsions, respiratory arrest, and permanent brain damage after elective surgery in healthy women. N Engl J Med 314:1529–1535, 1986

Arieff AI: Treatment of symptomatic hyponatremia: neither haste nor waste. Crit Care Med 19:748–751, 1991

Arieff AI, Schmidt RW: Fluid and electrolyte disorders and the central nervous system, in Clinical Disorders of Fluid and Electrolyte Metabolism, 3rd Edition. Edited by Maxwell MH, Kleeman CR. New York, McGraw-Hill, 1980, pp 1409–1480

Arieff AI, Llach F, Massry SG: Neurological manifestations and morbidity of hyponatremia: correlations with brain water and electrolytes. Medicine (Baltimore) 55:121–129, 1976

Arieff AI, Ayus JC, Fraser CL: Hyponatremia and death or permanent brain damage in healthy children. Br Med J 304:1218–1222, 1992

Arieti S: Interpretation of Schizophrenia, 2nd Edition. New York, Basic Books, 1974

Aronson PS: Energy-dependence of phlorizin binding to isolated renal microvillus membranes. J Membr Biol 42:81–98, 1978

Arslan Y, Burckhardt R, Jawaharal K, et al: Effects of narcotic analgesics on water and food intake in normal rats, in The Physiology of Thirst and Sodium Appetite. Edited by de Caro G, Epstein AN, Massi M. New York, Plenum, 1986, pp 527–534

Avruch J, Wallach DFH: Preparation and properties of plasma membrane and endoplasmic retuculum fragments from isolated rat fat cells. Biochim Biophys Acta 233:334–347, 1971

Aylward E, Walker E, Bettes B: Intelligence in schizophrenia: meta-analysis of the research. Schizophr Bull 10:430–458, 1984

Ayus JC, Krothapalli RK, Arieff AI: Changing concepts in treatment of severe symptomatic hyponatremia: rapid correction and possible relation to central pontine myelinolysis. Am J Med 78:897–901, 1985

Ayus JC, Krothapalli RK, Arieff AI: Treatment of symptomatic hyponatremia and its relation to brain damage. N Engl J Med 317:1190–1195, 1987

Ayus JC, Krothapalli RK, Arieff AI: Sexual difference in survival with severe symptomatic hyponatremia (Abstract). Kidney Int 33:181, 1988

Balagura S, Wilcox RH, Coscina DV: The effects of diencephalic lesions on food intake and motor activity. Physiol Behav 4:629–633, 1969

Baldessarini RJ, Frankenburg FR: Clozapine: a new antipsychotic agent. N Engl J Med 324:746–754, 1991

Barahal HS: Water intoxication in a mental case. Psychiatric Q 12:767–771, 1938

Barlow ED, De Wardener HE: Compulsive water drinking. Q J Med 28:235–258, 1959

Barta PE, Pearlson GD, Powers RE, et al: Auditory hallucinations and smaller superior temporal gyral volume in schizophrenia. Am J Psychiatry 147:1457–1462, 1990

Bartels M, Themelis J: Computerized tomography in tardive dyskinesia. Evidence of structural abnormalities in the basal ganglia system. Arch Psychiatr Nervenkr 233:371–379, 1983

Bartter FC, Schwartz WB: The syndrome of inappropriate secretion of antidiuretic hormone. Am J Med 42:790–806, 1967

Bates C, Horrobin DF, Ells K: Fatty acids in plasma phospholipids and cholesterol esters from identical twin concordant and discordant for schizophrenia. Schizophr Res 6:1–7, 1992

Bauer R: Zur pathologie und differentialdiagnose von "diabetes insipidus" und primrer polydipsie. Wiener Archiv Für Innere Medizin 11:201, 1925

Baylis PH, Robertson GL: The posterior pituitary: hormone secretion in health and disease, in Physiological Control of Vasopressin Secretion. Edited by Baylis PH, Padfield PL. New York, Marcel Dekker, 1985, pp 119–139

Beiser M, Erickson D, Fleming JA, et al: Establishing the onset of psychotic illness. Am J Psychiatry 150:1349–1354, 1993

Bello-Reuss EN, Grady TP, Mazumdar DC: Serum vanadium levels in chronic renal disease. Ann Intern Med 91:743, 1979

Berginer VM, Osimani A, Berginer J, et al: CT brain scan in acute water intoxication. J Neurol Neurosurg Psychiatr 48:841–846, 1985

Berl T: Treating hyponatremia: damned if we do and damned if we don't. Kidney Int 37:1006–1018, 1990a

Berl T: Treating hyponatremia: what is all the controversy about? Ann Intern Med 113:417–419, 1990b

Berl T, Schrier RW: Disorders of the water metabolism, in Renal and Electrolyte Disorders. Edited by Schrier RW. Boston, Little, Brown, 1986, pp 1–77

Berl T, Anderson RJ, Schrier RW: Clinical disorders of water metabolism. Kidney Int 10:117–132, 1976

Bernard C: Le cons de physiologie expérimentale appliquée à la médecine. Faites au Collage de France Cours du Semestre d'Eté. Paris, Bailliere, 1856

Besarab A, Silva P, Epstein FH: Multiple pumps for reabsorption by the perfused kidney. Kidney Int 10:147–153, 1976

Bhagavan BS, Wagner JA, Juanteguy J: Central pontine myelinolysis and medullary myelinolysis. Arch Pathol Lab Med 100:246–252, 1976

Bigelow LB, Berthot BD: The Psychiatric Symptom Assessment Scale (PSAS). Psychoparmacol Bull 25:168–179, 1989

Bilder RM, Mukherjee S, Reider RO, et al: Symptomatic and neuropsychological components of defect states. Schizophr Bull 11:409–419, 1985

Black RM: Diagnosis and management of hyponatremia. J Intensive Care Med 4:205–220, 1989

Black SL: Preoptic hypernatremia syndrome and the regulation of water balance in the rat. Physiol Behav 4:953–958, 1976

Blackwood DHR, Young AH, Muir WJ, et al: An MRI study in schizophrenia: relationships with structural imaging, evoked potentials and neuropsychological test results. Clin Neuropharmacol 15:114A, 1992

Blaine EH: Atrial natriuretic factor. Fed Proc 45:2360–2391, 1986

Blank DL, Wayner MJ: Lateral preoptic single unit activity: effects of various solutions. Physiol Behav 15:723–730, 1975

Blass EM, Epstein AN: A lateral preoptic osmosensitive zone for thirst in the rat. J Comp Physiol Psychol 76:378–394, 1971

Blass EM, Hall WG: Drinking termination: interactions between hydrational, orogastric and behavioral controls in rats. Psychol Rev 183:356–374, 1976

Blass EM, Hanson DG: Primary hyperdipsia in the rat following septal lesions. J Comp Physiol Psychol 70:87–93, 1970

Blass EM, AI Nussbaum, DG Hanson: Septal hyperdipsia: specific enhancement of drinking to angiotensin in rats. J Comp Physiol Psychol 87:422–439, 1974

Bleiler RE, Schedl HP: Creatinine excretion: variability and relationships to diet and body size. J Lab Clin Med 59:945–955, 1962

Bleuler E: Dementia Precox or the Group of Schizophrenias. New York, International Universities Press, 1950

Block ML, AE Fisher: Anticholinergic central blockade of salt-aroused and deprivation-induced thirst. Physiol Behav 5:525–527, 1970

Blotcky MJ, Grossman I, Looney JG: Psychogenic water intoxication: a fatality. Tex Med 76:58–59, 1980

Blum A: The possible role of tobacco cigarette smoking in hyponatremia of long-term psychiatric patients. JAMA 252:2864–2865, 1984

Blum A, Friedland GW: Urinary tract abnormalities due to chronic psychogenic polydipsia. Am J Psychiatry 140:915–916, 1983

Blum A, Tempey FW, Lynch WJ: Somatic findings in patients with psychogenic polydipsia. J Clin Psychiatry 44:55–56, 1983

Bogerts B: Zur neuropathologie der schizophrenien. Fortschr Neurol Psychiat 52:428–437, 1984

Bogerts B, Meertz E, Schonfeldt-Bausch R: Basal ganglia and limbic system pathology in schizophrenia. Arch Gen Psychiatry 42:784–791, 1985

Bogerts B, Lieberman JA, Ashtari M, et al: Hippocampus-amygdala volumes and psychopathology in chronic schizophrenia. Biol Psychiatry 33:236–246, 1993

Booth AG, Kenny AJ: A rapid method for the preparation of microvilli from rabbit kidney. Biochem J 142:575–581, 1974

Breier A, Buchanan RW, Elkashef AM, et al: Brain morphology and schizophrenia. Arch Gen Psychiatry 49:921–926, 1992

Bremner AJ, Regan A: Intoxicated by water. Polydipsia and water intoxication in a mental handicap hospital. Br J Psychiatry 158:244–250, 1991

Brenner RR: Effect of unsaturated acids on membrane structure and enzyme kinetics. Prog Lipid Res 23:69–96, 1984

Brimble MJ, Dyball REJ: Characterization of the responses of oxytocin- and vasopressin-secreting neurons in the supraoptic nucleus to osmotic stimulation. J Physiol (London) 271:253–271, 1977

Brown AC: Passive and active transport in Physiology and Biophysics, Vol. 2. Edited by Ruch TC, Patton HD. Philadelphia, Saunders, 1974, pp 820–842

Brown B, Grossman SP: Evidence that nerve cell bodies in the zona incerta influence ingestive behavior. Brain Res Bull 5:593–597, 1980

Brown RP, Kocsis JH, Cohen SK: Delusional depression and inappropriate antidiuretic hormone secretion. Biol Psychiatry 18:1059–1063, 1983

Brunner JE, Redmond JM, Haggar AM, et al: Central pontine myelinolysis after rapid correction of hyponatremia: a magnetic resonance imaging study. Ann Neurol 23:389–391, 1988

Brunner JE, Redmond JM, Haggar AM, et al: Central pontine myelinolysis and pontine lesions after rapid correction of hyponatremia: a prospective magnetic resonance imaging study. Ann Neurol 27:61–66, 1990

Buggy J: Drinking elicited by angiotensin or hypertonic stimulation of the rat antero-ventral third ventricle: single or separate neural substrates? Central Action of Angiotensin and Related Hormones. Edited by Buckley JP, Ferrario CM, Lokhandwala LF. New York, Pergamon, 1977

Buggy J, Johnson AK: Anteroventral third ventricle periventricular ablation: temporary adipsia and persisting thirst deficits. Neurosci Lett 5:177–182, 1977a

Buggy J, Johnson AK: Preoptic-hypothalamic periventricular lesions: thirst deficits and hypernatremia. Am J Physiol 233:R44–R52, 1977b

Bugle C, Andrew S, Heath J: Early detection of water intoxication. J Psychosoc Nurs Ment Health Serv 30:31–33, 1992

Bujis, RM: Vasopressin localization and putative functions in the brain, in Vasopressin: Principles and Properties. Edited by Gash DM, Boer GJ. New York, Plenum, 1987, pp 91–117

Burg MB, Grantham JJ, Abramov M, et al: Preparation and study of fragments of single rabbit nephrons. Am J Physiol 210:1293–1298, 1966

Burnell GM, Foster TA. Psychosis with low sodium syndrome. Am J Psychiatry 128:1313–1314, 1972

Cadnapaphornchai P, Boykin JL, Berl T, et al: Mechanism of effect of nicotine on renal water excretion. Am J Physiol 227:1216–1220, 1974

Cannon WB: The physiological basis of thirst. Proc R Soc Med, Series B, 90:283–301, 1919

Carpenter WT, Buchanan RW, Kirkpatrick B: The concept of the negative symptoms of schizophrenia, in Negative Schizophrenia: Symptoms, Pathophysiology and Clinical Implications. Edited by Tandon R, Greden JF. Washington, DC, American Psychiatric Press, 1991, pp 3–20

Casanova MF, Stevens JR, Kleinman JE: The Neuropathology of Schizophrenia. Old and New Findings, in New Biological Vistas on Schizophrenia. Edited by Lindenmayer JP, Kay SF. New York, Brunner/Mazel, 1992, pp 82–109

Castillo RA, Ray RA, Yaghmai F: Central pontine myelinolysis and pregnancy. Obstet Gynecol 73:459–461, 1989

Cheng J, Zikos D, Skopicki HA, Peterson DR, Fisher KA: Long-term neurologic outcome in psychogenic water drinkers with severe symptomatic hyponatremia: the effect of rapid correction. Am J Med 88:561–566, 1990

Choi DW: Ionic dependence of glutamate toxicity. J Neurosci 7:369–379, 1987

Chung H, Kluge R, Schrier RW, Anderson RJ: Clinical assessment of extracellular fluid volume in hyponatremia. Am J Med 83:905–908, 1987

Clardy JA, Hyde TM, Kleinman JE: Postmortem neurochemical and neuropathological studies in schizophrenia, in Schizophrenia: from mind to molecule. Edited by Andreasen NC. Washington, DC, American Psychiatric Press, 1994, pp 123–145

Clifford DB, Gado MH, Levy BK: Osmotic demyelination syndrome. Lack of pathologic and radiologic imaging correlation. Arch Neurol 46:343–347, 1989

Cluitmans FHM, Meinders AE: Management of severe hyponatremia: rapid or slow correction? Am J Med 88:161–166, 1990

Coburn PC, Stricker EM: Osmoregulatory thirst in rats after lateral preoptic lesions. J Comp Physiol Psychol 92:350–361, 1978

Coffman JA, Schwarzkopf SB: Temporal lobe asymmetry in schizophrenics demonstrated by coronal MRI brain scans. Schizophr Res 2:117, 1989

Cogan E, Debieve M, Pepersack T, et al: Natriuresis and atrial natriuretic factor secretion during inappropriate antidiuresis. Am J Med 84: 409–418, 1988a

Cogan E, Debieve M, Pepersack T, et al: Hyponatremia and atrial natriuretic peptide secretion in patients with vasopressin-induced antidiuresis. Am J Med 594–595, 1988b

Cohen BJ, Jordan MH, Chapin SD, et al: Pontine myelinolysis after correction of hyponatremia during burn resuscitation. J Burn Care Rehabil 12:153–156, 1991

Cooper SJ: Benzodiazepine and endorphinergic mechanisms related to salt and water intake, in The Physiology of Thirst and Sodium Appetite. Edited by de Caro G, Epstein AN, Massi M. New York, Plenum, 1986, pp 239–244

Copeland PM: Diuretic abuse and central pontine myelinolysis. Psychother Psychosom 52:101–105, 1989

Coppen A, Abou-Saleh M, Millin P, et al: Dexamethasone suppression test in depression and other psychiatric illness. Br J Psychiatry 142: 498–504, 1983

Corcoran AC: Electrometric urinometry: a note on comparative determinations of urinary osmolality and specific gravity. J Lab Clin Med 46:141–143, 1955

Costall B, Naylor RJ: Mesolimbic and extrapyramidal sites for the medication of stereotypied behavior patterns and hyperactivity by amphetamine and apomorphine in the rat, in Cocaine and Other Stimulants. Edited by Ellinwood EH, Kilby MM. New York, Plenum, 1977, pp 47–76

Crammer JL: Disturbances of water and sodium in a manic-depressive illness. Br J Psychiatry 149:337–345, 1986

Crayton JW, Meltzer HY: Degeneration and regeneration of motor neurons in psychotic patients. Biol Psychiatry 14:803–819, 1979

Crow TJ: Molecular pathology of schizophrenia: more than one disease process? Br Med J 280:66–68, 1980

Crow TJ: Schizophrenic deterioration. Br J Psychiatry 143:80–83, 1983

Crow TJ: The two-syndrome concept: origins and current status. Schizophr Bull 11:471–486, 1985

Crow TJ: Current view of the Type II Syndrome: significance of age of onset, intellectual impairment, and structural changes in the brain, in Negative Schizophrenia: Symptoms, Pathophysiology and Clinical Implications. Edited by Tandon R and Greden JF. Washington, DC, American Psychiatric Press, 1991, pp 163–171

Crow TJ, Mitchell WS: Subjective age in chronic schizophrenia: evidence for a subgroup of patients with defective learning capacity? Br J Psychiatry 126:360–363, 1975

Czech DA, Stein EA, Blake MJ: Naloxone-induced hypodipsia: a CNS mapping study. Life Sci 33:797–803, 1983

Daggett P, Deanfield J, Moss F: Neurological aspects of hyponatremia. Postgrad Med J 58:737–740, 1982

Daniel TO, Heinrich WL: Endocrine abnormalities and fluid and electrolyte disorders in Fluids and Electrolytes, 2nd Edition. Edited by Kokko JP, Tannen RL. Philadelphia, PA, WB Saunders, 1990, pp 830–870

Dashe AM, Cramm RE, Crist CA, et al: A water deprivation test for the differential diagnosis of polyuria. JAMA 185:639–703, 1963

Davidson C, Smith D, Morgan DB: Diurnal pattern of water and electrolyte excretion and body weight in idiopathic orthostatic hypotension. Am J Med 61:709–715, 1976

Davis JM: Dose equivalence of the antipsychotic drugs. J Psychiatr Res 2:65–69, 1974

Davis JRE, McNeill M, Millar JW: Iatrogenic water intoxication in psychogenic polydipsia. Scott Med J 26:148–150, 1981

Deas-Nesmith D, Brewerton TD: A case of Fluoxetine-responsive psychogenic polydipsia: A variant of obsessive-compulsive disorder? J Nerv Ment Dis 180:338–339, 1992

de Bold A: Atrial natriuretic factor: a hormone produced by the heart. Science 230:767–770, 1985

de Bold AJ: Atrial natriuretic factor. Fed Proc 45:2081–2132, 1986

de Bold AJ, Bornstein HB, Veress AT, et al: A rapid and potent natriuretic response to intravenous injections of atrial myocardial extracts in rats. Life Sci 28:89–94, 1981

de Caro G: Effects of peptides of the "Gut-Brain-Skin" triangle on drinking behavior of rats and birds, in The Physiology of Thirst and Sodium Appetite. Edited by de Caro G, Epstein AN, Massi M. New York, Plenum, 1986, pp 213–226

de Caro G, Micossi LG: Selective antidipsogenic effect of kassinin in Wistar rats, in The Physiology of Thirst and Sodium Appetite. Edited by de Caro G, Epstein AN, Massi M. New York, Plenum, 1986, pp 245–250

de Caro G, Epstein AN, Massi M (eds): The Physiology of Thirst and Sodium Appetite. New York, Plenum Press, 1986

Decaux G, Przedborski S, Soupart A: Lack of efficacy of phenytoin in the syndrome of inappropriate anti-diuretic hormone secretion of neurological origin. Postgrad Med 65:456–458, 1989

DeFronzo RA, Goldberg M, Agus AS: Normal diluting capacity in hyponatremic patients: reset osmostat or a variant of the syndrome of inappropriate antidiuretic hormone secretion. Ann Intern Med 84: 538–542, 1976

De La Rocha M, Aiken J, Lambert W: A psychiatric hospital ward for water intoxication. Biol Psychiatry 25:184A, 1989

DeLisi LE: The significance of age of onset for schizophrenia. Schizophr Bull 18:209–215, 1992

DeLisi LE, Dauphinais ID, Gershon ES: Perinatal complications and reduced size of brain limbic structures in familial schizophrenia. Schizophr Bull 14:185–191, 1988

Delva NJ, Crammer JL: Polydipsia in chronic psychiatric patients: Body weight and sodium. Br J Psychiatry 152:242–245, 1988

Delva NJ, Crammer JL, Jarzylo SV, et al: Osteopenia, pathological fractures, and increased urinary calcium excretion in schizophrenic patients with polydipsia. Biol Psychiatry 26:781–793, 1989

Delva NJ, Crammer JL, Lawson JS, et al: Vassopressin in chronic psychiatric patients with primary polydipsia. Br J Psychiatry 157:703–712, 1990

De Soto MF, Griffith SR, Katz EJ: Water intoxication associated with nephrogenic diabetes insipidus secondary to lithium: case report. J Clin Psychiatry 46:402–403, 1985

Devenport LD: Schedule-induced polydipsia in rats: adrenocortical and hippocampal modulation. J Comp Physiol Psychol 92:651–660, 1978

Devenport LD, Devenport JA, Holloway FA: Reward-induced stereotypy: modulation by the hippocampus. Science 212:1288–1289, 1981

De Wardener HE, Mills IH, Clapham WF, et al: Studies on the efferent mechanism of the sodium diuresis which follows the administration of intravenous saline in the dog. Clin Sci 21:249–258, 1961

DeWitt LD: CT follow-up in central pontine myelinolysis. Neurology 35:444, 1985

DeWitt LD, Buonanno FS, Kistler JP, et al: Central pontine myelinolysis: demonstration by nuclear magnetic resonance. Neurology 34:570–576, 1984

Dickoff DJ, Raps M, Yahr MD: Striatal syndrome following hyponatremia and its rapid correction: a manifestation of extrapontine myelinolysis confirmed by magnetic resonance imaging. Arch Neurology 45: 112–114, 1988

Díes F, Rangel S, Rivera A: Differential diagnosis between diabetes insipidus and compulsive polydipsia. Ann Intern Med 54:710–725, 1961

DiMaio VJM, DiMaio SJ: Fatal water intoxication in a case of psychogenic polydipsia. J Forensic Sci 25:332–335, 1980

Donnelly EF, Weinberger DR, Waldman IN, et al: Cognitive impairment associated with morphological brain abnormalities on computed tomography in chronic schizophrenic patients. J Nerv Ment Dis 168:305–308, 1980

Doucet A, Katz AI: Mineralocorticoid receptors along the nephron: [³H] aldosterone binding in rabbit tubules. Am J Physiol 241:F605–F611, 1981

Dourish CT: Dopaminergic involvement in the control of drinking behavior: a brief review. Prog Neuropsychopharmacol Biol Psychiatry 7: 487–493, 1983

Dubovsky SL, Grabon S, Berl T, Schrier RW: Syndrome of inappropriate secretion of antidiuretic hormone with exacerbated psychosis. Ann Intern Med 79:551–554, 1973

Dunn FL, Brennan TJ, Nelson AE, et al: The role of blood osmolality and volume in regulating vasopressin secretion in the rat. J Clin Invest 52:3212–3219, 1973

Ebstein W: Beiträge zur lehre vom diabetes insipidus. Dtsch Arch Klin Med 95:1, 1909

Edelman GM: Surface modulation in cell recognition and cell growth. Science 192:218–226, 1976

Edelman IS, Leibman J: Anatomy of body water and electrolytes. Am J Med 27:256–277, 1959

Edelman IS, Olney JM, James AH, et al: Body composition: studies in the human being by dilution principles. Science 115:447–454, 1952

Edelman IS, Leibman J, O'Meara MP: Interrelations between serum sodium concentration, serum osmolality and total exchangeable sodium, total exchangeable potassium and total body water. J Clin Invest 37:1236–1256, 1958

Edelson JT, Robertson GL: The effect of the cold pressor test on vasopressin secretion in man. Psychoneuroendocrinology 11:307–316, 1986

Edelstein SB, Breakefield XO: Human fibroblast cultures, in Physicochemical Methodologies and Psychiatric Research. Edited by Hanin I, Koslow SH. New York, Raven, 1980, pp 200–243

Editor: Water intoxication. Lancet 264:425–426, 1953

Elkashef AE, Buchanan R, Breier A, et al: Basal ganglia pathology in schizophrenia and tardive dyskinesia: an MRI quantitative study. Am J Psychiatry 151:15, 1994a

Elkashef AE, Issa F, Kirch DG, et al: Effects of water loading in schizophrenic patients with polydipsia-hyponatremia: an MRI pilot study. Schizophr Res 13:169–172, 1994b

Emsley R, Potgieter A, Taljaard F, et al: Water excretion and plasma vasopressin in psychotic disorders. Am J Psychiatry 146:250–253, 1989

Emsley RA, van der Meer H, Aalbers C, et al: Inappropriate antidiuretic state in long-term psychiatric inpatients. S Afr Med J 77:307–308, 1990

Emsley RA, Spangeberg JJ, Roberts MC, et al: Disordered water water homeostasis and cognitive impairment in schizophrenia. Biol Psychiatry 34:630–633, 1993

Epstein AN: Angiotensin in Encyclopedia of Neuroscience, Vol 1. Edited by Aldeman G. Boston, MA, Birkhauser, 1987, pp 49–51

Epstein AN, Teitelbaum P: Severe and persistent deficits in thirst produced by lateral hypothalamic damage, in Thirst in the Regulation of Body Water. Edited by Wayner MJ. Oxford, UK, Pergamon, 1964, pp 395–406

Epstein AN, Fitzsimons JT, Rolls SBJ: Drinking induced by injection of angiotensin into the brain of the rat. J Physiol (London). 210:457–474, 1970

Estol CJ, Faris AA, Martinez AJ, et al: Central pontine myelinolysis after liver transplantation. Neurology 39:493–498, 1989

Falk JL: Production of polydipsia in normal rats by an intermittent food schedule. Science 133:195–196, 1961

Falk JL, Tang M: Rapid sodium depletion and salt appetite induced by intraperitoneal dialysis, in Biological and Behavioral Aspects of Salt Intake. Edited by Kare MR, Fregley MJ, Bernard RA. New York, Academic Press, 1980, pp 205–220

Falkai P, Bogerts B: Cell loss in the hippocampus of schizophrenics. Eur Arch Psychiatry Clin Neurosci 236:154–161, 1986

Fambrough DM: The sodium pump becomes a family. Trends Neurosci 11:325–328, 1988

Farini A, Ceccaroni B: Influenza degli estratti ipofisari sull' eliminazione dell' acido ippurico. Gazz d osp 34:879, 1913

Feinberg I: Schizophrenia: caused by a fault in programmed synaptic elimination during adolescence. J Psychiatr Res 17:319–334, 1982

Feldberg W: Possible association of schizophrenia with a disturbance in prostaglandin metabolism: a physiological hypothesis. Psychol Med 6:359–369, 1976

Felix D, Gambino MC, Yong Y, et al: Angiotensin-sensitive sites in the central nervous system, in The Physiology of Thirst and Sodium Appetite. Edited by de Caro G, Epstein AN, Massi M. New York, Plenum, 1986, pp 135–140

Ferrier IN: Water intoxication in patients with psychiatric illness. Br Med J 291:1594–1596, 1985

Fichman MP, Kleeman CR, Bethune JE: Inhibition of antidiuretic hormone secretion by diphenylhydantoin. Arch Neurol 22:45–53, 1970

Fichman MP, Vorherr H, Kleeman CR, Teener N: Diuretic-induced hyponatremia. Ann Intern Med 75:853–863, 1971

Filuk PE, Miller MA, Dorsa DM, et al: Localization of messenger RNA encoding isoforms of the catalytic subunit of the (Na$^+$+ K$^+$)-ATPase in rat brain by in situ hybridization histochemistry. Neurosci Res Commun 5:155–162, 1989

Findlay JBC, Evans WH (eds): Biological Membranes, Oxford, UK, IRL Press, 1990

Finean JB, Coleman R, Green WA: Studies of isolated plasma membrane preparations. Ann NY Acad Sci 137:414–420, 1966

Fish B, Marcus J, Hans SL, et al: Infants at risk for schizophrenia: sequelae of a genetic neurodegenerative defect. Arch Gen Psychiatry 49: 221–235, 1992

Fisher AE: Relationship between cholinergic and other dipsogens in the central mediation of thirst, in Neuropsychology of Thirst: New Findings and Advances in Concepts. Edited by Epstein AN, Kissileff HR, Stellar E. New York, Wiley, 1973, pp 243–278

Fisher AE, Coury J: Cholinergic tracing of a central neural circuit underlying the thirst drive. Science 138:691–693, 1962

Fitzsimons JT: Drinking by nephrectomized rats injected with various substances. J Physiol (London) 155:563–579, 1961a

Fitzsimons JT: Drinking by rats depleted of body fluid without increase in osmotic pressure. J Physiol (London) 159:307–309, 1961b

Fitzsimons JT: Drinking caused by constriction of the vena cava. Nature 204:479–480, 1964

Fitzsimons JT: The role of renal thirst factor in drinking induced by extracellular stimuli. J Physiol (London) 201:349–368, 1969

Fitzsimons JT: The hormonal control of water and sodium intake, in Frontiers in Neuroendocrinology. Edited by Martini L, Ganong WF. New York, Oxford University Press, 1971a, pp 103–128

Fitzsimons JT: The physiology of thirst: a review of the extraneural aspects of the mechanisms of drinking, in Progress in Physiological Psychology, Vol 4. Edited by Stellar E, Sprague J. New York, Academic Press, 1971b, pp 119–201

Fitzsimons JT: The Physiology of Thirst and Sodium Appetite. Cambridge, MA, Cambridge University Press, 1979

Fitzsimons JT, Epstein AN, Johnson AK: Peptide antagonists of the renin-angiotensin system in the characterization of the receptors for angiotensin-induced thirst. Brain Res 153:319–331, 1978

Flear CTG, Gall GV, Burns J: Hyponatremia: mechanisms and management. Lancet 2(8236):26–31, 1981

Fleischhacker WW, Barnas C, Ledochowski M: Hyponatremia-induced organic mental disorder may mask paranoid schizophrenia. Biol Psychiatry 22:650–652, 1987

Flor-Henry P: The Cerebral Basis of Psychopathology. Littleton, MA, Wright PSG, 1983

Fluharty SJ: Cerebral prostaglandin biosynthesis and angiotensin-induced thirst. J Comp Physiol Psychol 95:915–923, 1981

Fluharty SJ, Epstein AN: Sodium appetite elicited by intracerebro-ventricular infusions of angiotensin II in the rat: synergistic interaction with systemic mineralocorticoids. Behav Neurosci 97:746–758, 1983

Folstein MF, Folstein SE, McHugh PR: Mini-Mental State: a practical method for grading the cognitive state of patients for the clinician. J Psychiatr Res 12:189–198, 1975

Forrest JN, Cox M, Hong C, et al: Superiority of demeclocyline over lithium in the treatment of chronic syndrome of inappropriate secretion of antidiuretic hormone. N Engl J Med 298:173–177, 1978

Fowler RC, Kronfol ZA, Perry PJ: Water intoxication, psychosis, and in appropriate secretion of antidiuretic hormone. Arch Gen Psychiatry 34:1097–1099, 1977

Fraser CL, Kucharczyk J, Arieff AI, et al: Sex differences result in increased morbidity from hyponatremia in female rats. Am J Physiol 256: R880–R885, 1989

Fraser D: Central pontine myelinolysis as a result of treatment of hyperemesis gravidarum. Case report. Br J Obstet Gynaecol 95: 621–623, 1988

Fricchoine G, Kelleher S, Ayyala M: Coexisting central diabetes insipidus and psychogenic polydipsia. J Clin Psychiatry 48:75–76, 1987

Friede R: The histochemical architecture of Ammons horn as it relates to its selective vulnerability. Acta Neuropathol 6:1–13, 1966

Ganong WF: Review of Medical Physiology. Los Altos, CA, Lange Medical Publications, 1971

Ganong WF: Sympathetic effects of renin secretion: mechanisms and physiological role. Adv Exp Med Biol 17:17–32, 1972

Ganong WF: The brain renin-angiotensin system. Annu Rev Physiol 46: 17–31, 1984

Ganten D, Hutchinson JS, Schelling P, et al: The isorenin-angiotensin system in extrarenal tissue. Clin Expt Pharmacol Physiol 3:103–126, 1976

Gardiner TW, Stricker EM: Hyperdipsia in rats after electrolytic lesions of nucleus medianus. Am J Physiol 248:R214–R223, 1985a

Gardiner TW, Stricker EM: Impaired drinking responses of rats with lesions of the nucleus medianus: circadian dependence. Am J Physiol 248:R224–R230, 1985b

Garrels JJ: Quantitative two-dimensional gel electrophoresis of proteins. Methods Enzymol 100:411–423, 1983

Gehi MM, Rosenthal RH, Fizette NB, et al: Psychiatric manifestations of hyponatremia. Psychosom 22:739–743, 1981

Gellai M, Allen DE, Beeuwkes R: Contrasting views on the action of atrial peptides: lessons from studies of conscious animals. Fed Proc 45:2387–2391, 1986

Gerard E, Healy ME, Hesselink JR: MR demonstration of mesencephalic lesions in osmotic demyelination syndrome: central pontine myelinolysis. Neuroradiology 29:582–594, 1987

Gerber O, Geller M, Stiller J, et al: Central pontine myelinolysis: resolution shown by computed tomography. Arch Neurol 12:116–118, 1983

Gibbs DM: Dissociation of oxytocin, vasopressin and corticotropin secretion during stress. Life Sci 35:487–491, 1984

Giller EL: The use of fibroblast cultures in neuropsychiatric disorders, in Physicochemical Methodologies and Psychiatric Research. Edited by Hanin I, Koslow SH. New York, Raven, 1980, pp 245–256

Gillum DM, Linas SL: Water intoxication in a psychotic patient with normal renal water excretion. Am J Med 77:773–774, 1984

Gleadhill IC, Smith TA, Yium JJ: Hyponatremia in patients with schizophrenia. South Med J 75:426–428, 1982

Glowinski J, Herve D, Tassin JP: Heterologous regulation of receptors on target cells of dopamine neurons in the frontal cortex, nucleus accumbens, and striatum. Ann N Y Acad Sci 537:112–123, 1988

Glusac E, Patel H, Josef NC, et al: Polydipsia and hyponatremia induced by multiple neuroleptics but not molindone. Can J Psychiatry 35:268–269, 1990

Gocht A, Colmant HJ: Central pontine and extrapontine myelinolysis: a report of 58 cases. Clin Neuropathol 6:262–270 1987

Godleski LS, Vieweg WVR, Yank GR: Prevalence of polyuria among chronically psychotic men. Psychiatr Med 6:114–120, 1988

Godleski LS, Vieweg WVR, Leadbetter RA, et al: Day-to-day care of chronic schizophrenic patients subject to water intoxication. Annals of Clinical Psychiatry 1:179–185, 1989

Goebel HH, Herman-Ben Zur P: Central pontine myelinolysis: a clinical and pathological study of 10 cases. Brain 95:495–504, 1972

Gold PW, Robertson GL, Post R, et al: The effect of lithium on the osmoregulation of arginine vasopressin secretion. J Clin Endocrinol Metab 56:295–299, 1983b

Golden CJ, Moses JA, Zelazowski R, et al: Cerebral ventricular size and neuropsychological impairment in young chronic schizophrenics: measurement by the standardized Luria-Nebraska neuropsychological battery. Arch Gen Psychiatry 37:619–623, 1980

Golden CJ, MacInnes WD, Ariel RN, et al: Cross-validation of the ability of the Luria-Nebraska neuropsychological battery to differentiate chronic schizophrenics with and without ventricular enlargement. J Consult Clin Psychol 50:87–95, 1982

Goldman JE, Horoupian DS. Demyelination of the lateral geniculate nucleus in central pontine myelinolysis. Ann Neurol 9:185–189, 1981

Goldman M: A rational approach to disorders of water balance in psychiatric patients. Hosp Community Psychiatry 42:488–494, 1991

Goldman MB, Janecek HM: Is compulsive drinking a compulsive behavior? a pilot study. Biol Psychiatry 29:503–505, 1991

Goldman MB, Luchins DJ: Demeclocycline improves hyponatremia in chronic schizophrenics. Biol Psychiatry 20:1149–1155, 1985

Goldman MB, Luchins DJ: Prevention of episodic water intoxication with target weight procedure. Am J Psychiatry 144:365–366, 1987

Goldman MB, Luchins DJ, Robertson GL: Mechanisms of altered water metabolism in psychotic patients with polydipsia and hypo-natremia. N Engl J Med 318:397–403, 1988

Goldman MB, Luchins DJ, Robertson GL: Treatment of hyponatremia secondary to water overload. Lancet 1:328–329, 1989

Goldman MB, Marks RC, Blake L, et al: Estimating daily urine volume in psychiatric patients: empiric confirmation. Biol Psychiatry 31:1228–1231, 1992

Goldman MB, Blake L, Marks RC, et al: Association of nonsuppression of cortisol on the DST with primary polydipsia in chronic schizophrenia. Am J Psychiatry 150:653–655, 1993

Goldman MB, Christiansen B, Gaskill MB, et al: Hippocampal lesions enhance vasopressin response to stress. Presented at the annual meeting of the American Psychiatric Association, Philadelphia, PA, May 1994

Goldman MB, Robertson GL, Hedeker D, et al: The influence of polydipsia on water excretion in hyponatremic polydipsic schizophrenic patients. J Clin Endocrinol Metab (in press a)

Goldman MB, Robertson GL, Hedeker D: Oropharyngeal regulation of water balance in polydipsic schizophrenics. Clin Endocrinol (in press b)

Goldstein CS, Braunstein S, Goldfarb S: Idiopathic syndrome of inappropriate antidiuresis secretion possibly related to advanced age. Ann Intern Med 99:185–188, 1983

Goldstein G, Zubin J, and Pogue-Geile M: Hospitalization and the cognitive deficits of schizophrenia: the influences of age and education. J Nerv Ment Dis 179:202–206, 1991

Goldstein JA: Therapeutic lessons from a family practitioner. Therapaeia 73–84, 1981

Goldstein JA: Captopril in the treatment of psychogenic polydipsia. J Clin Psychiatry 47:99, 1986

Gonick HC, Kramer HJ, Paul W, et al: Circulating inhibitor of sodium-potassium-activated adenosine triphosphatase after expansion of extracelluler fluid volume in rats. Clin Sci Mol Med 53:329–334, 1977

Goodwin FK, Jamison KR: Manic-depressive illness. New York, Oxford University Press, 1990

Grafton ST, Bahls FH, Bell KR. Acquired focal dystonia following recovery from central pontine myelinolysis. J Neurol Neurosurg Psychiatry 51:1354–1355, 1988

Granstrom E: Biochemistry of the eicosanoids: cyclooxygenase and lipooxygense products of polyunsaturated fatty acids, in Lipids in Modern Nutrition. Edited by Horisberger M, Bracco U. New York, Raven, 1987, pp 59–66

Green R, Giebisch G: Ionic requirements of proximal tubual sodium transport. I. Bicarbonate and chloride. Am J Physiol 229:1205–1215, 1975

Greenberg WM, Shah PJ, Vakharia M: Anorexia nervosa/bulemia and central pontine myelinolysis. Gen Hosp Psychiatry 14:357–358, 1992

Grishman CM, Barnett RE: The role of lipid-phase transitions in the regulation of the (sodium + potassium) adenosine triphosphatase. Biochemistry 12:2635–2637, 1973

Gross JB, Bartter FC: Effects of prostaglandins E_1, A_1, and F_2 on renal handling of salt and water. Am J Physiol 225:218–225, 1973

Gross PA, Pehrisch H, Rasher W: Pathogenesis of clinical hyponatremia: observations of vasopressin and fluid intake in 100 hyponatremic medical patients. Eur J Clin Invest 17:123–129, 1987

Gross S, Bell RD: Central pontine myelinolysis and rapid correction of hyponatremia. Tex Med 78:59–60, 1982

Grossman SP: Eating or drinking elicited by direct adrenergic or cholinergic stimulation of hypothalamus. Science 132:301–302, 1960

Grossman SP: Direct adrenergic and cholinergic stimulation of hypothalamic mechanisms. Am J Physiol 202:872–882, 1962a

Grossman SP: Effects of adrenergic and cholinergic blocking agents on hypothalamic mechanisms. Am J Physiol 202:1230–1236, 1962b

Grossman SP: Thirst and Sodium Appetite. San Diego, CA, Academic Press, 1990, pp 1–10

Grossman SP, Grossman L: Parametric study of the regulatory capabilities of rats with rostromedial zona incerta lesions: responsiveness to hypertonic saline and polyethylene glycol. Physiol Behav 21:432–440, 1978

Grossman SP, Dacey D, Hallaris AE, et al: Aphagia and adipsia after preferential destruction of nerve cell bodies in the hypothalamus. Science 202:557–559, 1978

Gruzelier J, Seymore K, Wilson L, et al: Impairments on neuropsychological tests of temporohippocampal and frontohippocampal functions and word fluency in remitting schizophrenia and affective disorders. Arch Gen Psychiatry 45:623–629, 1988

Gur RE: MRI and cognitive behavioral function in schizophrenia. J Neural Transm 36:13–22, 1992

Gutman Y, Krausz M: Drinking induced by dextran and histamine: relation to kidneys and renin. Eur J Pharmacol 23:256–263, 1973

Habener JF, Dashe AM, Solomon DH: Response of normal subjects to prolonged high fluid intake. J Appl Physiol 19:134–136, 1964

Hagenfeldt L, Venizelos N, Bjerkenstedt L, et al: Decreased tyrosine transport in fibroblasts from schizophrenic patients. Life Sci 41:2749–2757, 1987

Haibach H, Ansbacher LE, Dix JD: Central pontine myelinolysis: a complication of hyponatremia or of therapeutic intervention? J Forensic Sci 32:444–451, 1987

Haller EW, Wakerly BJ: Electrophysiological studies of paraventricular and supraoptic neurons recorded in vitro from slices of rat hypothalamus. J Physiol (London) 302:347–362, 1980

Hantman D, Rossier B, Zohlman R, Schrier RW: Rapid correction of hyponatremia in the syndrome of inappropriate antidiuretic hormone: an alternative treatment to hypertonic saline. Ann Intern Med 78:870–875, 1973

Hariprasad MK, Eisinger RP, Nadler IM, et al: Hyponatremia in psychogenic polydipsia. Arch Intern Med 140:1639–1642, 1980

Harris VJ: The dexamethasone suppression test and residual schizophrenia. Am J Psychiatry 142(5):659–660, 1985

Harris WE, Stahl WL: Protein-lipid interactions of the $(Na^+ + K^+)$-ATPase, in The Sodium Pump. Edited by Glynn I, Ellory C, Cambridge, MA, Company of Biologists, 1985, pp 73–76

Harrison RB, Ramchandani P, Allen JT: Psychogenic polydipsia: unusual cause for hydronephrosis. Am J Rad 133:327–328, 1979

Hazratji SMA, Kim RC, Lee SH, et al: Evolution of pontine and extrapontine myelinolysis. J Comput Assist Tomogr 7:356–361, 1983

Heaton RK, Drexler M: Clinical neuropsychological findings in schizophrenia and aging, in Schizophrenia and Aging. Edited by Miller NE, Cohen GD. New York, Guilford Press, 1987, pp 145–161

Heckers S, Heinsen H, Heinsen Y, et al: Cortex, white matter, and basal ganglia in schizophrenia: a volumetric postmortem study. Biol Psychiatry 29:556–566, 1991

Hellerstein DJ, Meehan B: Outpatient group therapy for schizophrenic substance abusers. Am J Psychiatry 144:1337–1339, 1987

Helwig FC, Schutz CB, Curry DE: Water intoxication: report of a fatal human case, with clinical, pathologic, and experimental studies. JAMA 104:1569–1575, 1935

Hennessy JW, Grossman SP, Kanner MA: A study of the etiology of the hyperdipsia produced by coronal knife cuts in the posterior hypothalamus. Physiol Behav 18:73–80, 1977

Hernandez-Peon R, Chavez-Ibarra G, Morgane PJ, et al: Cholinergic pathways for sleep, alertness and rage in the limbic midbrain circuit. Acta Neurol Lat Am 8:93–96, 1962

Herrera VL, Emanuel JR, Ruiz-Opazo N, et al: Three differentially expressed ($Na^+ + K^+$)-ATPase alpha units isoforms: structural and functional implications. J Cell Biol 104:1855, 1987

Hickey RC, Hare K: The renal excretion of chloride and water in diabetes insipidus. J Clin Invest 23:768–775, 1944

Hieber V, Siegel GJ, Fink DJ, et al: Differential distribution of ($Na^+ + K^+$)-ATPase isoforms in the central nervous system. Cell Mol Neurobiol 11:253–262, 1991

Hitzemann R, Hirschowitz J, Graver D: Membrane abnormalities in the psychoses and affective disorders. Psychiatry Res 18:319–326, 1984

Hobson JA, English JT: Self-induced water intoxication: Case study of a chronically schizophrenic patient with physiological evidence of water retention due to inappropriate release of antidiuretic hormone. Ann Intern Med 58:324–332, 1963

Hoffman WE, Phillips MI: Regional study of cerebral ventricle sensitive sites of angiotensin II. Brain Res. 108:59–73, 1976

Horrobin DF: Essential Fatty Acids, Prostaglandins and Schizophrenia in Psychiatry: A World Perspective, Vol 2. Edited by Stephanis CN, Soldatos CR, Raburilas AD. Amersterdam, Exerpta Medica, 1990, pp 140–144

Horrobin DF: The relationship between schizophrenia and essential fatty acid and eicosenoid metabolism. Prostaglandins Leukot Essent Fatty Acids 46:71–77, 1992

Horrobin DF, Manku MS, Morse-Fisher N, et al: Essential fatty acids in plasma phospholipids in schizophrenics. Biol Psychiatry 25:562–568, 1989

Horrobin DF, Manku MS, Hillman S, et al: Fatty acid levels in the brains of schizophrenics and normal controls. Biol Psychiatry 30:795–805, 1991

Horrobin DF, Skinner F, Glen I: Membrane essential fatty acids (EFAs) show a biphasic distribution in schizophrenics with predominantly positive or predominantly negative symptoms (abstract). Schizophr Res 6:135, 1992

Hoskins RG: Schizophrenia from a physiologic point of view. Ann Intern Med 30:123–140, 1933

Hoskins RG, Sleeper FH: Organic functions in schizophrenia. Arch Neurol Psychiatry 30:123–140, 1933

Hosutt JA, Rowland N, Stricker NE: Hypotension and thirst in rats after isoproterenol treatment. Physiol Behav 21:593–598, 1978

Hosutt JA, Rowland N, Stricker EM: Impaired drinking responses of rats with lesions of the subfornical organ. C Comp Physiol Psychol 95: 104–113, 1981

Hsu YM, Guidotti G: Rat brain has the alpha 3 form of the $(Na^+ + K^+)$-ATPase. Biochemistry 28:569–573, 1989

Huang Y, Mogenson G: Neural pathways mediating drinking and feeding in rats. Exp Neurol 37:269–286, 1972

Illowsky BP: Psychiatric aspects of CNS myelinolysis. Presented at the 143rd annual meeting of the American Psychiatric Association, New York, May 1990

Illowsky BP, Kirch DG: Polydipsia and hyponatremia in psychiatric patients. Am J Psychiatry 145:675–783, 1988

Illowsky BP, Laureno R: Encephalopathy and myelinolysis after rapid correction of hyponatremia. Brain 110:855–867, 1987

Ingram DA, Traub M, Kopelman PG, et al: Brain-stem auditory evoked responses in diagnosis of central pontine myelinolysis. J Neurol 233:23–24, 1986

Inoue K, Tadai T, Kamimura H, et al: The syndrome of self-induced water intoxication in psychiatric patients. Folia Psychiatr Neurol Jpn 39:121–128, 1985

Iovino M, Steardo L: The role of the septal area in the regulation of drinking behavior and plasma ADH secretion, in The Physiology of Thirst and Sodium Appetite. Edited by de Caro G, Epstein AN, Massi M. New York, Plenum, 1986, pp 367–374

Jacobi W, Winkler H: Encephalographische studies au chronisch schizophrenen. Archiv Psychiatr Nevenkrankheiten 81:299–332, 1927

Jernigan TL, Zisook S, Heaton RK, et al: Magnetic resonance imaging abnormalities in lenticular nuclei and cerebral cortex in schizophrenia. Arch Gen Psychiatry 48:881–890, 1991

Jeste DV, Lohr JB: Hippocampal pathological findings in schizophrenia: a morphometric study. Arch Gen Psychiatry 46:1019–1124, 1989

Johnson AK, Buggy J: A critical analysis of the site of action for the dipsogenic effect of angiotensin II, in Central Actions of Angiotensin and Related Hormones. Edited by Buckley JP, Ferrario CM. New York, Pergamon, 1977, pp 357–385

Johnson AK, Buggy J: Periventricular preoptic-hypothalamus is vital for thirst and normal water economy. Am J Physiol 234:R122–R127, 1978

Johnson AK, Epstein AN: The cerebral ventricles as the avenue for the dipsogenic action of intracranial angiotensin. Brain Res 86:399–418, 1975

Johnson AK, Robinson MM, Mann JFE: The role of the renal renin-angiotensin system in thirst, in The Physiology of Thirst and Sodium Appetite. Edited by de Caro G, Epstein AN, Massi M. New York, Plenum, 1986, pp 161–180

Johnstone EC, Crow TJ, Frith CD, et al: Cerebral ventricular size and cognitive impairment in chronic schizophrenia. Lancet 2:924–926, 1976

Johnstone EC, Crow TJ, Frith CD, et al: The dementia of dementia praecox. Acta Psychiatr Scand 57:305–324, 1978

Johnstone EC, Owens DGC, Gold A, et al: Institutionalization and the defects of schizophrenia. Br J Psychiatry 139: 195–203, 1981

Johnstone EC, Owens DGC, Crow TJ, et al: Temporal lobe structure as determined by nuclear magnetic resonance in schizophrenia and bipolar affective disorder. J Neurol Neurosurg Psychiatry 52:736–741, 1989

Jones BD: Psychosis associated with water intoxication: psychogenic polydipsia or concomitant dopaminergic supersensitivity disorders? Lancet 2:519–520, 1984

Jorgensen PL: Sodium and potassium ion pump in kidney tubules. Physiol Rev 60:864–917, 1980

Jos CJ: Generalized seizures from self-induced water intoxication. Psychosomatics 25:153–157, 1984

Jos CJ, Evenson RC, Mallya AR: Self-induced water intoxication: a comparison of 34 cases with matched controls. J Clin Psychiatry 47: 368–370, 1986

Jose CJ, Evenson RC: Antecedents of self-induced water intoxication. J Nerv Ment Dis 168:498–500, 1980

Jose CJ, Perez-Cruet J: Incidence and morbidity of self-induced water intoxication in state mental hospital patients Am J Psychiatry 136: 221–222, 1979

Jose CJ, Barton JL, Perez-Cruet J: Hyponatremic seizures in psychiatric patients. Biol Psychiatry 14:839–843, 1979

Kachanoff R, Leveille R, McLelland JP, et al: Schedule-induced behavior in humans. Physiol Behav 11(3):395–398, 1973

Kaiya H, Horrobin DF, Manku MS, et al: Essential and other fatty acids in plasma in schizophrenics and normal individuals from Japan. Biol Psychiatry 30:357–362, 1991

Kandt RS, Heldrich FJ, Moser HW: Recovery from probable central pontine myelinolysis associated with Addison's disease. Arch Neurol 40:118–119, 1983

Kane J, Honigfeld G, Singer J, et al: Clozaril Collaboration Study group. Clozapine for the treatment-resistant schizophrenic: a double-blind comparison with chlorpromazine. Arch Gen Psychiatry 45:789–796, 1988

Karp BI, Laureno R: Pontine and extrapontine myelinolysis: a neurological disorder following rapid correction of hyponatremia. Medicine 72(6):359–373, 1993

Kathol RG, Wilcos JA, Turner RD, et al: Pharmacologic approaches to psychogenic polydipsia: case reports. Prog Neuropsychopharmacol Biol Psychiat 10:95–100, 1986

Katz AI: Renal Na-K-ATPase: its role in tubular sodium and potassium transport. Am J Physiol 242:F207–F219, 1982

Katzman R, Clasen R, Klatzo I, et al: Report of joint committee for stroke resources, IV: brain edema in stroke. Stroke 8:512–540, 1977

Kay SR, Fizbein A, Opler L: Positive and Negative Syndrome Scale (PANSS) for schizophrenia. Schizophr Bull 13:261–276, 1987

Keefe RSE, Mohs RC, Losonczy MF, et al: Characteristics of very poor outcome schizophrenia. Am J Psychiatry 144:889–895, 1987

Kelsoe JR, Cadet JL, Pickar D, et al: Quantitative neuroanatomy in schizophrenia. Arch Gen Psychiatry 45:533–541, 1988

Kenney NJ: Suppression of water intake by the E prostaglandins, in The Physiology of Thirst and Sodium Appetite. Edited by de Caro G, Epstein AN, Massi M. New York, Plenum, 1986, pp 227–238

Kenney NJ, Moe KE, Skoog KM: The antidipsogenic action of peripheral prostaglandin E2. Pharmacol Biochem Behav 15:263–269, 1981

Khamnei AK: Psychosis, inappropriate antidiuretic hormone secretion, and water intoxication (Letter). Lancet 1:963, 1984

Kimble DP: Hippocampus and internal inhibition. Psychol Bull 70: 285–295, 1968

Kimelberg HK: The influence of membrane fluidity on activity of membrane-bound enzymes, in Cell Surface Reviews, Vol. 3. Edited by Poste G, Nicolson GL. Amsterdam, Elsevier/North Holland, 1977, pp 205–293

King BM, Grossman SP: Response to glucoprivic and hydrational challenges by normal and hypothalamic hyperphagic rats. Physiol Behav 18:463–473, 1977

Kinne R, Schwartz IL: Isolated membrane vesicles in the evaluation of the nature, localization and regulation of renal transport processes. Kidney Int 14:547–556, 1978

Kinsella JL, Aronson PS: Properties of the Na^+-H^+ exchanger in renal microvillus membrane vesicles. Am J Physiol 238:F461–F469, 1980

Kirch DG, Weinberger DR: Anatomical neuropathology in schizophrenia: post mortem findings, in Handbook of Schizophrenia, The Neurology of Schizophrenia. Edited by Nasrallah HA, Weinberger DR. Amsterdam, Elsevier, 1986, pp 325–349

Kirch DG, Bigelow LB, Weinberger DR: Polydipsia and chronic hyponatremia in schizophrenic inpatients. J Clin Psychiatry 46:179–181, 1985

Kirch DG, Elkashef A, Suddath RL, et al: The neuroanatomy of polydipsia-hyponatremia. 1992 CME Syllabus & Proceedings Summary, 145th Annual Meeting of the American Psychiatric Association, Washington, DC, May 2–7, 1992, p 193

Kirschenbaum MA: Renal disease: practical diagnosis. Boston, MA, Houghton Mifflin, 1978

Kishimoto T, Hirai M, Ohsawa H, et al: Manners of arginine vasopressin secretion in schizophrenic patients—with reference to the mechanism of water intoxication. Jpn J Psychiatry Neurol 43:161–169, 1989

Kissileff HR: Food associated drinking in the rat. J Comp Physiol Psychol 67:284–300, 1969

Kissileff HR, Epstein AN: Exaggerated prandial drinking in the 'recovered lateral' rat without saliva. J Comp Physiol Psychol 67:301–308, 1969

Kleinschmidt-Demasters BK, Norenberg MD: Rapid correction of hyponatremia causes demyelination: relation to central pontine myelinolysis. Science 211:1068–1080, 1981

Kleinschmidt-DeMasters BK, Norenberg MD: Neuropathologic observations in electrolyte-induced myelinolysis in the rat. J Neuropath Exp Neurol 41:67–80, 1982

Klonoff EA, Moore DJ: Compulsive polydipsia presenting as diabetes insipidus: a behavioral approach. J Behav Ther Exp Psychiatry 15: 353–358, 1984

Kluver H, Bucy PC: Preliminary analysis of the temporal lobes in monkeys. Archives of Neurology and Psychiatry 42:979–1000, 1939

Koci TM, Chiang F, Chow P, et al: Thalamic extrapontine lesions in central pontine myelinolysis. Am J Neuroradiol 11:1229–1233, 1990

Koczapski AB, Millson RC: Individual differences in serum sodium levels in schizophrenic men with self-induced water intoxication. Am J Psychiatry 146:1614–1615, 1989

Koczapski A, Ibraheem S, Paredes J, et al: Diurnal variations in hyponatremia and body weight in chronic schizophrenics with self-induced water intoxication. J Clin Invest 8:A86, 1985

Koczapski AB, Millson RC, MacEwan GW, et al: Estimation of fluid intake in polydipsic schizophrenics. Paper presented at the Second Biannual International Congress on Schizophrenia Research, San Diego, CA, April 1989

Kofoed L, Kania J, Walsh T, Atkinson RM: Outpatient treatment of patients with substance abuse and coexisting psychiatric disorders. Am J Psychiatry 143:867–872, 1986

Kozlowski S, Drzewiecki K: The role of osmoreceptors in portal circulation in control of water intake in dogs. Acta Physiol Pol 24:325–330, 1973

Kraly FS: Abdominal vagotomy inhibits osmotically induced drinking in the rat. J Comp Physiol Psychol 92:999–1013, 1978

Kraly FS: Histamine plays a role in drinking elicited by eating in the rat, in The Physiology of Thirst and Sodium Appetite. Edited by de Caro G, Epstein AN, Massi M. New York, Plenum, 1986, pp 295–299

Kramer DS, Drake ME Jr: Acute psychosis, polydipsia, and inappropriate secretion of antidiuretic hormone. Am J Med 75:712–714, 1983

Kraepelin, E: Dementia Praecox and Paraphrenia. Edited by Robertson GM. Huntington, NY, Krieger, 1919

Kucharczyk J, Mogenson GJ: Separate lateral hypothalamic pathways for extracellular and intracellular thirst. Am J Physiol 228:295–301, 1975

Kühn ER: Cholinergic and adrenergic release mechanisms for vasopressin in the male rat: a study with injections of neurotransmitters and blocking agents into the third ventricle. Neuroendocrinology 16:255–264, 1974

Kurokawa K: Effects of hormones on renal function, in Textbook of Nephrology, Vol 1, 2nd Edition. Edited by Massry SG, Glassock RJ. Baltimore, MD, Williams & Wilkins, 1989, pp 160–167

Kushnir M, Schattner A, Ezri T, et al: Case report: schizophrenia and fatal self-induced water intoxication with appropriately-diluted urine. J Med Sci 300:385–387, 1990

Lakowicz JR: Principles of fluorescence spectroscopy, New York, Plenum, 1983

Lapierre E, Berthot BD, Gurvitch M, et al: Polydipsia and hyponatremia in psychiatric patients: challenge to creative nursing care. Arch Psychiatric Nurs 4:87–92, 1990

Laureno R: Central pontine myelinolysis following rapid correction of hyponatremia. Ann Neurol 13:232–242, 1983

Laureno R, Karp BI: Pontine and extrapontine myelinolysis following rapid correction of hyponatremia. Lancet 1:1439–1441, 1988

Lawson WB: Polyuria and schizophrenia. Psychiatry Res 17:331–332, 1986

Lawson WB, Hagstrom EC, Walter GF: Salt preference in desalivate rats. Physiol Behav 12:733–739, 1974

Lawson WB, Karson CN, Bigelow LB: Increased urine volume in chronic schizophrenic patients. Psychiatry Res 14:323–331, 1985

Lawson WB, Williams B, Pasion R: Effects of captopril on psychosis and disturbed water regulations. Psychopharmacol Bull 24:176–178, 1988

Lawson WB, Kirch DG, Shelton R, et al: Computer tomographic and endocrine findings in schizophrenic patients with hyponatremia (Abstract #95). Biol Psychiatry 29:46A, 1991

Leadbetter RA, Spears N, Shutty MS: Influence of clozapine on polydipsia and hyponatremia. Paper presented at the annual meeting of the American Psychiatric Association, San Francisco, CA, May 1993

Leadbetter RA, Spears N, Shutty MS: Impact of clozapine on polydipsia/hyponatremia. 1994 CME Syllabus & Proceedings Summary, 147th Annual Meeting of the American Psychiatric Association, Philadelphia, PA, May 1994, p 180

Leaf A: Regulation of intracellular fluid volume and disease. Am J Med 49:291–295, 1970

Lee HS, Kwon KY, Alphs LD et al: Effect of clozapine on psychogenic polydipsia in chronic schizophrenia. J Clin Psychopharmacol 11:222–223, 1991

Lee MC, Thrasher TN, Ramsay DJ: Is angiotensin essential in drinking induced by water deprivation and caval ligation. Am J Physiol 240:R75–R80, 1981

Leenen FH, Stricker EM, McDonald RJH, et al: Relationship between increase in plasma renin activity and drinking following different types of dipsogenic stimuli, in Control Mechanisms of Drinking. Edited by Peters G, Fitzsimons JT, Peters-Haefeli L. New York, Springer-Verlag, 1975, pp 84–88

Lehr D, Mallow J, Kurkowski M: Copious drinking and simultaneous inhibition of urine flow elicited by beta-adrenergic stimulation and contrary effect of alpha-adrenergic stimulation. J Pharmacol Exp Therap 158:150–163, 1967

Lehr D, Goldman HW, Casner P: Renin-angiotensin role in thirst: paradoxical enhancement of drinking by angiotensin converting enzyme inhibition. Science 182:1031–1034, 1973

Lehr D, Goldman HW, Casner P: Evidence against the postulated role of the renin-angiotensin system in putative renin-dependent drinking responses, in Control Mechanisms of Drinking. Edited by Peters G, Fitzsimons JT, Peters-Haefeli L. New York, Springer-Verlag, 1975, pp 79–83

Leibowitz SF: Histamine: A stimulatory effect on drinking in the rat. Brain Res 63:440–444, 1973a

Leibowitz SF: Histamine: Modification of behavioral and physiological components of body fluid homeostasis, in Histamine Receptors. Edited by Yellin TO. New York, Spectrum Press, 1979, pp 219–253

Leibowitz SF: Neurochemical systems of the hypothalamus, in Handbook of the Hypothalamus, Vol 3, "Behavioral Studies of the Hypothalamus." Edited by Morgane PJ, Panksepp J. New York, Marcel Dekker, 1980, 299–437

Levine S, McManus BM, Blackbourne BD, et al: Fatal water intoxication, schizophrenia, and diuretic therapy for systemic hypertension. Am J Med 82:153–155, 1987

Levinsky NG: Fluid and electrolytes, in Harrison's Principles of Internal Medicine, 12th Edition. Edited by Wilson JD, Braunwald E, Isselbacher KJ, et al. New York: McGraw-Hill, 1991, pp 178–184

Levitt RA, Fisher AE: Cholinergic substrate for drinking in the rat. Psychol Rev 29:431–448, 1971

Lightman SL, Forsling M: Evidence for dopamine and an inhibitor of vasopressin release in man. J Clin Endocrinol Metab 12:39–46, 1980

Liljestrand G, Zotterman Y: The water taste in mammals. Acta Physiol Scand 32:291–303, 1954

Lind RW, Johnson AK: Subfornical organ-median preoptic connections and drinking and pressor responses to angiotensin II. J Neurosci 2:1043–1051, 1982

Lohr JB, Kuczenski R, Bracha HS, et al: Increased indices of free radical activity in the cerebrospinal fluid of patients with tardive diskinesia. Biol Psychiatry 28:535–539, 1990

Losonczy MF, Song IS, Mohs RC, et al: Correlates of lateral ventricular size in chronic schizophrenia: II: Biologic measures. Am J Psychiatry 143:1113–1117, 1986

Lowry OH, Passoneau JV (eds): A Flexible System of Enzyme Analysis. New York, Academic Press, 1972

Luchins DJ: A possible role of hippocampal dysfunction in schizophrenic symptomatology. Biol Psychiatry 28:87–91, 1990

Luchins DJ, Goldman MB, Lieb M, et al: Repetitive behaviors in chronically institutionalized schizophrenic patients. Schizophr Res 8: 119–123, 1992a

Luchins DJ, Goldman MB, Lieb M, et al: Repetitive behaviors in chronic schizophrenia, in 1992 CME Syllabus & Proceedings Summary, 145th Annual Meeting of the American Psychiatric Association, Washington, DC, May 2–7, 1992b, p 193

Lyons M: Animal models of mania and schizophrenia, in Behavioral Models in Psychopharmacology: Theoretical, Industrial, and Clinical Perspectives. Edited by Willner P. London, Cambridge University Press, 1991, pp 253–310

Lyon M, Ludzik T, Lawson WB, et al: Potential animal of increased ETOH intake in schizophrenia: prenatal d-amphetamine exposure vs. pair-feeding control conditions (abstract). Schizophr Res 9:243, 1993

MacDonald HL, Bell BA, Smith MA, et al: Correlation of human NMR T1 values measured in vivo and brain water content. Br J Radiol 59: 355–357, 1986

MacLennan AJ, Maier SF: Coping and stress-induced potentiation of stimulant sterotypy in the rat. Science 219:1091–1093, 1983

Maddison S, Wood RJ, Rolls ET, et al: Drinking in the rhesus monkey: peripheral factors. J Comp Physiol Psychol 94:365–374, 1980

Maffly RH, Leaf A: The potential of water in mammalian tissues. J Gen Physiol 42:1257, 1959

Mahadik SP: Gangliosides, new generation neuroprotective agents, in Emerging Strategies in Neuroprotection. Edited by Morangos P, Lal H. Boston, MA, Burkhauser, 1992, pp 187–223

Mahadik SP, Karpiak SE: Gangliosides in treatment of neural injury and disease. Drug Development Research 15:337–360, 1988

Mahadik SP, Tamir H, Rapport MM: Macromolecular composition and functional organization of synaptic structures, in Advances in Neurochemistry. Edited by Agranff B, Aprison M. New York, Plenum, 1978, pp 99–163

Mahadik SP, Mukherjee S, Laev H, et al: Abnormal growth of skin fibroblasts from schizophrenic patients. Psychiatry Res 37:309–320, 1991

Mahadik SP, Bharucha VA, Stadlin A, et al: Loss and recovery of a+ and a isozymes of (Na^++ K^+)-ATPase in cortical focal ischemia: GM1 ganglioside protects plasma membrane structure and function. J Neurosci Res 32:209–220, 1992

Malmo RB, Malmo HP: Responses of lateral preoptic neurons in the rat to hypertonic sucrose and NaCl. EEG Clin Neurophysiol 45:401–408, 1979

Mandell AJ, Mersol-Sabbot I, Mandell MP: Psychological disturbance and water retention. Arch Gen Psychiatry 10:513–518, 1964

Mangiapane ML, Simpson JB: Subfornical organ lesions reduce the pressor effect of systemic angiotensin II. Neuroendocrinology 31:380–384, 1980

Mani R, Laureno R: Neuro-ophthalmic features of central pontine myelinolysis, in Neuro-opthalmology Now! Edited by Smith JL. New York, Field, Rich & Associates, 1986, pp 323–327

Mann JFE, Johnson AK, Ganten D: Plasma angiotensin II: Dipsogenic levels and angiotensin-generating capacity of renin. Am J Physiol 238:372–377, 1980

Manning PT, Schwartz D, Katsube NC, et al: Vasopressin-stimulated release of atriopeptin: endocrine antagonists in fluid homeostasis. Science 229:395–397, 1985

Manschreck TC, Maher BA, Rucklos ME, et al: Disturbed voluntary motor activity in schizophrenic disorder. Psychiatr Med 12:429–432, 1982

Maraganore DM, Folger WN, Swanson JW, et al: Movement Disorders as sequelae of central pontine myelinolysis: report of three cases. Movement Dis 7:142–148, 1992

Marshall JF, Richardson JS, Teitelbaum P: Nigrostriatal bundle damage and the lateral hypothalamic syndrome. J Comp Physiol Psychol 87:808–830, 1974

Masiak MJ, Naylor MD: The needs: fluids and electrolytes in Fluids and electrolytes through the life cycle. Edited by Masiak MJ, Naylor MD, Hayman LL. Norwalk, CT, Appleton-Century-Crofts, 1985, pp 3–26

Masterson E, O'Shea B: Smoking and malignancy in schizophrenia. Br J Psychiatry 145:429–432, 1984

Mata M, Fink DJ, Gainer H, et al: Activity-dependent energy metabolism in rat posterior pituitary primarily reflects sodium pump activity. J Neurochem 34:213–215, 1980

McColl P, Kelly C: A misleading case of central pontine myelinolysis: risk factors for psychiatric patients. Br J Psychiatry 160:550–552, 1992

McCormick W, Danneel C: Central pontine myelinolysis. Arch Int Med 119:444–478, 1967

McFarland DJ, Rolls BJ: Suppression of feeding by intracranial injections of angiotensin. Nature 236:172–173, 1972

McGowan MK, Brown B, Grossman SP: Depletion of neurons from lateral preoptic area impairs drinking to various dipsogens. Physiol Behav 43:815–822, 1988a

McGowan MK, Brown B, Grossman SP: Lesions of the MPO or AV3V: influences on fluid intake. Physiol Behav 42:331–342, 1988b

McKinley MJ: Volume regulation of antidiuretic hormone secretion, in Current Topics in Neuroendocrinology. Edited by Ganten D, Pfaff D. Berlin, Springer-Verlag, 1985, pp 61–100

McKinley MJ, Denton DA, Weisinger RS: Sensors for antidiuresis in thirst-osmoreceptors or CSF sodium detectors. Brain Res 141:89–103, 1978

McKinley MJ, Denton DA, Leksell LA, et al: Osmoregulatory thirst in sheep is disrupted by ablation of the anterior wall of the optic recess. Brain Res 236:210–215, 1982

McKinley MJ, Denton DA, Park RG, et al: Cerebral involvement in dehydration-induced natriuresis. Brain Res 236:340–347, 1983

McNally R, Calamari J, Hansen P, et al: Behavioral treatment of psychogenic polydipsia. J Behav Ther Exp Psychiatry 19:57–61, 1988

Mednick SA: Breakdown in individuals at high risk for schizophrenia: possible redispositional perinatal factors. Ment Hyg 54:50–63,

Mendelson J: Feedback control of hypothalamic drinking. Physiol Behav 5:779–781, 1970

Messert B, Orrison WW, Hawkins MJ, et al: Central pontine myelinolysis: considerations on etiology, diagnosis, and treatment. Neurology 29:147–160, 1979

Meyer DK, Peskar B, Tauchmann U, et al: Potentiation and abolition of the increase in plasma renin activity seen after hypotensive drugs in rats. Eur J Pharmacol 16:278–282, 1971

Meynert T: Psychiatrie. Vienna, W. Braumuller, 1884

Miller GM, Baker HL, Okazaki H, et al: Central pontine myelinolysis and its imitators: MR findings. Radiology 168:795–802, 1988

Miller M, Moses AM: Clinical states due to alteration of ADH release and action, in Proceedings of the Neurohypophysis International Conference. Basel, Karger, 1977, pp 15–166

Miller NE: Motivational effects of brain stimulation and drugs. Fed Proc 19:846–853, 1960

Miller NE: Chemical coding of behavior in the brain. Science 148:328–338, 1965

Miller NE, Sampliner RI, Woodrow P: Thirst reducing effects of water by stomach fistula versus water by mouth, measured by both a consummatory and an instrumental response. J Comp Physiol Psychol 50: 1–5, 1957

Millson RC, Koczapski AB, Cook M, et al: Self-induced water intoxication: the patients speak (abstract). Schizophr Res 2:167, 1989

Millson RC, Koczapski AB, Cook MI, et al: A survey of patient attitudes toward self-induced water intoxication. Can J Psychiatry 37:46–47, 1992

Millson RC, Smith AP, Koczapski AB, et al: Self-induced water intoxication treated with group psychotherapy. Am J Psychiatry 150:825–826, 1993

Mion CC, Andreasen NC, Arndt S, et al: MRI abnormalities in tardive dyskinesia. Psychiatric Research: Neuroimaging 40:157–166, 1992

Miselis RR: The efferent projections of the subfornical organ of the rat: a circumventricular organ within a neural network subserving water balance. Brain Res 230:1–23, 1981

Miselis RR, Shapiro RE, Hand PJ: Subfornical organ efferents to neural systems for control of body water. Science 205:1022–1023, 1979

Mitsui T, Ogura T, Ota Z, et al: Effects of dopamine on renal receptors for arginine vasopressin. Res Commun Chem Pathol Pharmacol 76: 131–141, 1992

Mogenson GJ: Stability and modification of consummatory behavior elicited by electrical stimulation of the hypothalamus. Physiol Behav 6:255–260, 1971

Mogenson GJ, Stevenson JAF: Drinking induced by electrical stimulation of the lateral hypothalamus. Exp Neurol 17:119–127, 1967

Mogenson GJ, Gentil CG, Stevenson JAF: Feeding and drinking elicited by low and high frequencies of hypothalamic stimulation. Brain Res 33:127–133, 1971

Moore FD: Determination of total body water and solids with isotopes. Science 104:157–160, 1946

Moran J, Blass EM: Inhibition of drinking by septal stimulation in rats. Physiol Behav 17:23–27, 1976

Morel F: Sites if hormone action in the mammalian nephron. Am J Physiol 240:F159–F164, 1981

Morgane PJ: Alterations in feeding and drinking behavior of rats with lesions in the globi pallidi. Am J Physiol 201:420–428, 1961

Moriwaka F, Tashiro K, Maruo Y, et al: MR imaging of pontine and extrapontine myelinolysis. J Comput Assist Tomogr 12:446–449, 1988

Morlan L, Rodriguez E, Gonzalez J, et al: Central pontine myelinolysis following correction of hyponatremia: MRI diagnosis. Eur Neurol 30:149–152, 1990

Morris JF, Chapman DB, Sokol HW: Anatomy and function of the classic vasopressin-secreting hypothalamus-neurohypophysial system, in Vasopressin: Principles and Properties. Edited by Gash DM, Boer GJ. New York, Plenum, 1987, pp 1–89

Moskowitz DW: Functional obstructive uropathy: a significant factor in the hyponatremia of psychogenic polydipsia. J Urol 147:1611–1613, 1992

Mukherjee S, Reddy S, Schnur D: Developmental model of negative syndromes in schizophrenia, in Negative Schizophrenic Syndromes. Edited by Greden J, Tandon, R. Washington, DC, American Psychiatric Press, 1991, pp 175–185

Murer H, Hopfer U, Kinne R: Sodium/proton antiport in brush-border-membrane vesickes isolated from rat small intestine and kidney. Biochem J 154:597–604, 1976

Myers RD: Emotional and autonomic responses following hypothalamic chemical stimulation. Can J Psychol 18:6–14, 1964

Narayanan S, Appleton HD: Creatinine: a review. Clin Chem 26:1119–1126, 1980

Narins RG: Therapy of hyponatremia. N Eng J Med 314:1573–1574, 1986

Nasrallah HA, Skinner TE, Schmalbrock, et al: [1]H nuclear magnetic resonance spectroscopy of the hippocampus in schizophrenia. 1992 CME Syllabus & Proceedings Summary, 145th Annual Meeting of the American Psychiatric Association, Washington, DC, May 1992, p 227

Neuringer M, Connor WE, Lin DS, et al: Biochemical and functional effects of prenatal and post-natal n-3 fatty acid deficiency on retina and brain in rhesus monkey. Proc Natl Acad Sci U S A 83:4021–4025, 1986

Nicolaidis S: Neurophysiologie sensorielle. Réponses des unités osmosensible hypothalamique aux stimulation saslines et aqueuses de la lange. C R Acad Sci Hebd Seances Acad Sci D 267:2352–2355, 1968

Nicolaidis S, Fitzsimons JT: La dépendance de la prise d'eau induite par l'angiotensine II envers la fonction vasomotrice locale chez le rat. C R Acad Sci Hebd Seances Acad Sci D 281:1417–1420, 1975

Nicolaidis S, Jeulin AC: Converging projections of hydromineral imbalances and hormonal co-action upon neurons surrounding the anterior wall of the third ventricle. J Physiol (Paris) 79(6):406–415, 1984

Nicolaidis S, Rowland N: Long-term self-intravenous drinking in the rat. J Comp Physiol Psychol 87:1–15, 1974

Nicolaidis S, Rowland N: Systemic versus oral and gastro-intestinal metering of fluid intake, in Control Mechanisms of Drinking. Edited by Peters G, Fitzsimons JT, Peters-Haefeli L. New York, Springer, 1975, pp 14–21

Nishikawa T, Tsuda A, Tanaka M, et al: Naloxone attenuates drinking behavior in schizophrenic patient displaying self-induced water intoxication. Clin Neuropharmacol 15:310–314, 1992

Nixon RA: Dr. Nixon replies (Letter). Am J Psychiatry 139:1525, 1982

Nixon R, Rothman J, Chin W: Demeclocycline in the prophylaxis of self-induced water intoxication. Am J Psychiatry 139:828–830, 1982

Norenberg M, Papendick R: Chronicity of hyponatremia as a factor in experimental myelinolysis. Ann Neurol 15:544–547, 1984

Nörgaard JP, Pedersen EB, Djurhuus JC: Diurnal antidiuretic hormone levels in enuretics. J Urol 134:1029–1031, 1985

Norgren R: The central organization of the gustatory and visceral afferent systems in the nucleus of the solitary tract, in Brain Mechanisms of Sensation. Edited by Katsuki Y, Norgren R, Sato M. New York, Wiley, 1981, pp 143–160

O'Kelly LI, Falk LJ, Flint D: The effects of preloads of water and sodium chloride on voluntary water intake of thirsty rats. J Comp Physiol Psychol 47:7–13, 1954

Ogilvie AD, Croy MF: Clozapine and hyponatraemia (Letter). Lancet 340:672, 1992

Oh MS, Uribarri J, Barrido D, et al: Case report: danger of central pontine myelinolysis in hyotonic dehydration and recomendation for treatment. Am J Med Sci 296:41–43, 1989

Okeda R, Kitano M, Sawabe M, et al: Distribution of demyelinating lesions in pontine and extrapontine myelinolysis-3 autopsy cases including one case devoid of central pontine myelinolysis. Acta Neuropathol (Berl) 69:259–266, 1986

Olson K, Rundgren M: Inefficiency of isoprenaline to induce drinking in the goat. Acta Physiol Scand 93:553–559, 1975

Olson SC, Nasrallah HA, Coffman JA, et al: CT and MRI abnormalities in schizophrenia: Relationship with negative symptoms, in Negative Schizophrenia: Symptoms, Pathophysiology and Clinical Implications. Edited by Tandon R, Greden JF. Washington, DC, American Psychiatric Press, 1991, pp 148–160

Oomura Y, Ono T, Ooyama H, et al: Glucose- and osmosensitive neurons in the rat hypothalamus. Nature 222:3282–3284, 1969

Owens DGC, Johnstone EC: The disabilities of chronic schizophrenia—their nature and the factors contributing to their development. Br J Psychiatry 136:384–395, 1980

Owens DGC, Johnstone EC, Frith CD: Spontanious involuntary disorders of movement. Arch Gen Psychiatry 39:452–461, 1982

Owens DGC, Johnstone E, Crow TJ, et al: Lateral ventricular size in schizophrenia: relationship to the disease process and its clinical manifestations. Psychol Med 15:27–41, 1985

Pavalonis D, Shutty M, Hundley P, et al: Behavioral intervention to reduce water intake in the syndrome of psychosis, intermittent hyponatremia, and polydipsia. J Behav Ther Exp Psychiatry 23:51–57, 1992

Peces R, Ablanedo P, Alvarez J: Central pontine and extrapontine myelinolysis following correction of severe hyponatremia. Nephron 49:160–163, 1988

Peck JW: Discussion: Thirst(s) resulting from bodily water imbalances, in The Neuropsychology of Thirst. Edited by Epstein AN, Kissileff HR, Stellar E. New York, Wiley, 1973, pp 99–112

Peck JW, Novin D: Evidence that osmoreceptors mediating drinking in rabbits are in the lateral preoptic area. J Comp Physiol Psychol 74: 134–140, 1971

Peh LH, Devan GS, Low BL: A fatal case of water intoxication in a schizophrenic patient. Br J Psychiatry 156:891–894, 1990

Perfumi M, de Caro G, Massi M, et al: Inhibition of Ang II-induced drinking by dermorphin given into the SFO or into the lateral ventricle of intact or of SFO lesioned rats, in The Physiology of Thirst and Sodium Appetite. Edited by De Caro G, Epstein AN, Massi M. New York, Plenum, 1986, pp 257–264

Peters JP, Van Slyke DD: Quantitative Clinical Chemistry: Interpretations, Vol. 1. Baltimore, MD, Williams & Wilkins, 1946

Peterson DT, Marshall WH: Polydipsia and inappropriate secretion of antidiuretic hormone associated with hydrocephalus. Ann Intern Med 83:675–676, 1975

Pettegrew JW, Keshavan MS, Kaplan DB, et al: Alterations in brain high-energy phosphate and membrane phospholipid metabolism in first episode, drug-naive schizophrenics. Arch Gen Psychiatry 48:563–568, 1991

Pfohl B, Winokur G: The evolution of symptoms in institutionalized hebephrenic/catatonic schizophrenics. Br J Psychiatry 141:567–572, 1982

Phillips MI: Angiotensin in the brain. Neuroendocrinology 25:354–377, 1978

Phillips MI: Functions of angiotensin in the central nervous system. Annu Rev Physiol 25:413–435, 1987

Phillips MI, Hoffman WE: Sensitive sites in the brain for the blood pressure and drinking responses to angiotensin, in Central Actions of Angiotensin and Related Hormones. Edited by Buckley JP, Ferrario CM. New York, Pergamon, 1977, pp 325–356

Phillips PA, Rolls BJ, Ledingham GG, et al: Reduced thirst after water deprivation in healthy elderly men. N Engl J Med 311:753–759, 1984b

Price BH, Mesulam MM: Behavioral manifestations of central pontine myelinolysis. Arch Neurology 44:671–673, 1987

Quillen EW, Cowley AW: Influence of volume changes on osmolality-vasopressin relationships in conscious dogs. Am J Physiol 244: H73–H79, 1983

Rabe A, Haddad RK: Acquisition of 2-way shuttle box avoidance after selective hippocampal lesions. Physiol Behav 4:391–393, 1969

Radford EP: Factors modifying water metabolism in rats fed dry diets. Am J Physiol 196:1098–1108, 1959

Ragavan V, Verbalis J, Wood M, et al: Psychogenic polydipsia and hyponatremia: evidence for a reset osmostat. Presented at the 7th International Congress of Endocrinology, Quebec, Canada, May 1984

Ragland RL, Duffis AW, Gendelman S, et al: Central Pontine myelinolysis with clinical recovery: MRI documentation. J Comput Assist Tomogr 13:316–318, 1989

Ramsay DJ, Thrasher TN: Hyperosmotic and hypervolemic thirst, in The Physiology of Thirst and Sodium Appetite. Edited by de Caro G, Epstein AN, Massi M. New York, Plenum, 1986, pp 83–96

Ramsay DJ, Rolls BJ, Wood RJ: Thirst following water deprivation in dogs. J Physiol (London) 232:93–100, 1977

Raskind M: Psychosis, polydipsia, and water intoxication: report of a fatal case. Arch Gen Psychiatry 30:112–114, 1974

Raskind MA, Orenstein H, Christopher TG: Acute psychosis, increased water ingestion, and inappropriate antidiuretic hormone secretion in psychiatric patients. Am J Psychiatry 132:907–910, 1975

Raskind MA, Weitzman RE, Orenstein H, et al: In antidiuretic hormone elevated in psychosis: a pilot study. Biol Psychiatry 13:385–390, 1978

Raskind MA, Courtney N, Murburg M, et al: Antipsychotic drugs and plasma vasopressin in normals and acute schizophrenic patients. Biol Psychiatry 22:453–462, 1987

Raz S, Raz N: Structural brain abnormalities in the major psychoses: a quantitative review of the evidence from computerized imaging. Psychol Bull 108:93–108, 1990

Reddy R, Mahdik SP, Murthy JN, et al: Enzymes of antioxidant defense system in chronic schizophrenic patients. Biol Psychiatry 30:409–412, 1991

Reichardt M: Der diabetes insipidus, symptom einer geisteskrankheit? Arb a d psychiat Klin zu Wurzburg 2:49, 1908

Reisbick S, Neuringer M, Hasnain R, et al: Polydipsia in rhesus monkeys deficient in omega-3 fatty acids. Physiol Behav 47:315–323, 1990

Reisbick S, Neuringer N, Connor WE, et al: Increased intake of water and NaCl solutions in omega-3 fatty acid deficient monkeys. Physiol Behav 49:1139–1146, 1991

Reisbick S, Neuringer M, Connor WE, et al: Postnatal deficiency of omega-3 fatty acids in monkeys: fluid intake and urine concentration. Physiol Behav 51:473–479, 1992

Rendell M, McGrane D, Cuesta M: Fatal compulsive water drinking. JAMA 240:2557–2559, 1978

Resnick ME, Patterson C: Coma and convulsions due to compulsive water drinking. Neurology 19:1125–1126, 1969

Reveley AM, Reveley MA: Cerebral ventricular size in twins discordant for schizophrenia. Lancet 1:540–551, 1982

Richardson DB, Mogenson GJ: Water intake elicited by injections of angiotensin II into the preoptic area. Am J Physiol 240:R70–R74, 1981

Richter CP: Increased salt appetite in adrenalectomized rats. Am J Physiol 115:155–161, 1936

Riggs J, Schochet SJ. Osmotic stress, osmotic myelinolysis, and oligodendrocyte topography. Arch Pathol Lab Med 113:1386–1388, 1989

Riggs AT, Dysken MW, Kim WS, et al: A review of disorders of water homeostasis in psychiatric patients. Psychosomatics 32:133–148, 1991

Ripley TL, Millson RC, Koczapski AB: Self-induced water intoxication and alcohol abuse. Am J Psychiatry 146:102–103, 1989

Rippe DJ, Edwards MK, D'Amour PG, et al: MR imaging of central pontine myelinolysis. Journal of Computed Assisted Tomography 11:724–726, 1987

Robbins TW, Koob GF: Selective disruption of displacement behavior by lesions of the mesolimbic dopamine system. Nature 285:409–412, 1980

Roberts GW: Schizophrenia as an anomaly of development of cerebral asymmetry. Arch Gen Psychiatry 46:1145–1150, 1989

Robertson GL: Physiology of ADH secretion. Kidney Int 32 (suppl 21):S20–S26, 1987

Robertson GL, Athar S: The interaction of blood osmolality and blood volume in regulating plasma vasopressin in man. J Clin Endocrinol Metab 42:613–620, 1976

Robertson GL, Mahr EA, Athar S, Sinha T: Development and clinical application of a new method for the radioimmunoassay of arginine vasopressin in human plasma. J Clin Invest 52:2340–2352, 1973

Robertson GL, Shelton RL, Athar S: The osmoregulation of vasopressin. Kidney Int 10:25–37, 1976

Rolls BJ, Jones BP, Fallows DJ: A comparison of the motivational properties induced by intracranial angiotensin and water deprivation. Physiol Behav 9:777–782, 1972

Rolls BJ, Wood RJ, Stevens RM: Effects of palatability on body fluid homeostasis. Physiol Behav 20:15–19, 1978

Rolls BJ, Wood R , Rolls ET, et al: Thirst following water deprivation in humans. Am J Physiol 239:R476–R482, 1980a

Rolls BJ, Wood RJ , Rolls ET: Thirst: the initiation, maintenance, and termination of drinking, in Progress in Psychobiology and Physiological Psychology. Edited by Sprague JM, Epstein AN. New York, Academic Press, 1980b, pp 263–321

Rolls BJ, Phillips PA, Ledfingham JGG, et al: Human thirst: the controls of water intake in healthy men, in The Physiology of Thirst and Sodium Appetite. Edited by De Caro G, Epstein AN, Massi M. New York, Plenum, 1986, pp 521–526

Rosenbaum JF, Rothman JS, Murray GB: Psychosis and water intoxication. J Clin Psychiatry 40:287–291, 1979

Rosenbloom S, Buchholz D, Kumar AJ, et al: Evolution of central pontine myelinolysis on CT. Am J Neuroradiol 5:110–112, 1984

Rotrosen J, Wolkin A: Phospolipid and prostaglandin hypotheses of schizophrenia, in Psychopharmacology: The Third Generation of Progress. Edited by Meltzer HY. New York, Raven, 1987, pp 759–764

Rowe JW, Kilgore A, Robertson GL: Evidence in man that cigarette smoking induces vasopressin release via an airway-specific mechanism. J Clin Endocrinol Metab 51:170–172, 1980

Rowland N: Comparison of the suppression by naloxone of water intake induced in rats by hyperosmolality, hypovolemia and angiotensin. Pharmacol Biochem Behav 16:87–91, 1982

Rowland N, Nicolaidis S: Metering of fluid intake and determinants of ad libitum drinking in rats. Am J Physiol 231:1–8, 1976

Rowland N, Grossman L, Grossman SP: Zona incerta lesions: regulatory drinking deficits to intravenous NaCl, angiotensin but not to salt in the food. Physiol Behav 23:745–750, 1979

Rowntree LG: The water balance of the body. Physiol Rev 2:116–169, 1922

Rowntree LG: Water intoxication. Arch Intern Med 32:158–174, 1923

Russell PJD, Abdelaal AE, Mogenson GJ: Graded levels of hemorrhage, thirst and angiotensin II in the rat. Physiol Behav 15:117–119, 1975

Sachs G: Ion pumps in the renal tubule. Am J Physiol 233:F359–F365, 1977

Saffer D, Metcalf M, Coppen A: Abnormal dexamethasone suppression test in type II schizophrenia. Br J Psychiatry 147:721–723, 1985

Sanchez-Olea R, Pasantes-Morales H, Schousboe A: Neurons respond to hypo-osmotic conditions by an increase in intracellular free calcium. Nuerochem Res 18:147–152, 1993

Sandifer MG: Hyponatremia due to psychotropic drugs. J Clin Psychiatry 44:301–303, 1983

Sanger DJ: Opiates and ingestive behavior, in Theory in Psychopharmacology, Vol. 2. Edited by Cooper SJ. London, Academic Press, 1983, pp 75–113

Santy PA, Schwartz MB: Hyponatremia disguised as an acute manic episode. Hosp Community Psychiatry 34:1156–1157, 1983

Saper CB, Levisohn D: Afferent connections of the median preoptic nucleus in the rat: anatomical evidence for a cardiovascular integrative mechanism in the anteroventral third ventricular (AV3A) region. Brain Res 288:21–31, 1983

Sapolski RM, Plotski PM: Hypercortisolism and its possible neural bases. Biol Psychiatry 27:937–952, 1990

Schäfer EA, Herring PT: The action of pituitary extracts upon the kidney. Proc R Soc Lond B Biol Sci 77:571–572, 1906

Scheibel AB, Kovelman JA: Disorientation of pyramidal cell and its processes in the schizophrenia patient. Biol Psychiatry 16:101–102, 1981

Schmidt-Nielsen B, Schmidt-Nielsen K, Haupt TR, et al: Water balance of the camel. Am J Physiol 185:185–194, 1956

Schneider JW, Mercer RW, Gilmore-Herbert M, et al: Tissue specificity localization in brain and cell-free translation of mRNA encoding the A3 isoform of (Na$^+$+ K$^+$)–ATPase. Proc Natl Acad Sci U S A 85:284–288, 1988

Schnur DB, Wirkowski E, Reddy R, et al: Cognitive impairments in schizophrenic patients with hyponatrenia. Biol Psychiatry 33:836–838, 1993

Schrier RW: Appropriate versus inappropriate secretion of antidiuretic hormone. West J Med 121:62–64, 1974

Schroth G: Clinical and CT confirmed recovery from central pontine myelinolysis. Neuroradiology 26:149–151, 1984

Schuurmans-Stekhoven F, Bonting SL: Transport adenosine triphosphatases: properties and functions. Physiol Rev 61:1–76, 1981

Schwartz WB, Bennett W, Curelop S, et al: A syndrome of renal sodium loss and hyponatremia probably resulting from inappropriate secretion of antidiuretic hormone. Am J Med 23:529–542, 1957

Schwartz WB, Tassel D, Bartter FC: Further observations on hyponatremia and renal sodium loss probably resulting from inappropriate secretion of antidiuretic hormone. N Engl J Med 262:743–748, 1960

Schwob JE, Johnson AK: Evidence for the involvement of the renin-angiotensin system in isoproterenol dipsogenesis (Abstract). Neurosci Abstr 1:467, 1975

Sclafani A, Berner CN, Maul G: Feeding and drinking pathways between medial and lateral hypothalamus. J Comp Physiol Psychol 85:29–51, 1973

Sebastian CS, Bernardin AS: Comparison of enalapril and captropril in the management of self-induced water intoxication. Biol Psychiatry 27:787–790, 1990

Seeman MV: Schizophrenia in women and men, in Treating Chronically Mentally Ill Women. Edited by Bachrach LL, Nadelson CC. Washington, DC, American Psychiatric Press, 1988

Setler PE: The role of catecholamines in thirst, in The Neuropsychology of Thirst. Edited by Epstein AN, Kissileff HR, Stellar E. New York, Wiley, 1975, pp 279–290

Shade RE, Share L: Vasopressin release during nonhypotensive hemorrhage and angiotensin infusions. Am J Physiol 228:149–154, 1975

Shah PJ, Greenberg WM: Polydipsia with hyponatremia in a state hospital population. Hosp Community Psychiatry 43:509–511, 1992

Share L: The role of vasopressin in cardiovascular regulation. Physiol Rev 68:1248–1284, 1988

Shelton RC, Weinberger DR: X-ray computerized tomography studies, in The Neurology of Schizophrenia. Edited by Nasrallah H, Weinberger DR. Amsterdam, Elsevier, 1986, pp 207–250

Shen WW, Sata LS: Hypothalamic dopamine receptor supersensitivity? A pilot study of self-induced water intoxication. Psychiatr J Univ Ott 8:154–158, 1983

Shenn WW, Sata LS: Self-induced water intoxication and hyperdopaminergic state. Am J Psychiatry 141:1305–1306, 1984

Shenton ME, Kikinis R, Jolesz FA, et al: Abnormalities of the left temporal lobe and thought disorder in schizophrenia: a quantitative magnetic resonance imaging study. N Engl J Med 327:604–612, 1992

Shevitz SA, Jameison RC, Petrie WM, et al: Compulsive water drinking treated with high dose propanolol. J Nerv Ment Dis 168:246–248, 1980

Shull GE, Greeb J, Lingrel JB: Molecular cloning of three distinct forms of the (Na^++ K^+)-ATPase alpha-subunit from rat brain. Biochemistry 25:8125–8132, 1986

Shutty MS, Leadbetter RA: Salt appetite in patients who exhibit the syndrome of psychosis, intermittent hyponatremia, and polydipsia. Am J Psychiatry 150:674–675, 1993

Shutty MS Jr, Hundley PL, Leadbetter RA, et al: Development and validation of a behavioral observation measure for the syndrome of psychosis, intermittent hyponatremia, and polydipsia. J Behav Ther Exp Psychiatry 23:213–219, 1992

Shutty M, Briscoe L, Sautter S, et al: Neuropsychiatric manifestations of hyponatremia in chronic schizophrenic patients with psychosis, intermittent hyponatremia and polydipsia. Schizophr Res 10:125–130, 1993

Shutty MS, Sona Y, McCulley KM: Behavioral assessment: polydipsia in schizophrenia. 1994 CME Syllabus & Proceedings Summary, 147th Annual Meeting of the American Psychiatric Association, Philadelphia, PA, May 21–26, 1994, p 179

Siesjo BK, Bengtsson F: Calcium fluxes, calcium antagonists, and calcium-related pathology in brain ischemia, hypoglycemia, and spreading depression: a unifying hypothesis. J Cereb Blood Flow Metab 9: 127–140, 1989

Silbert PL, Knezevic WV, Peake HID, et al: Behavioural changes due to pontine and extrapontine myelinolysis. Med J Aust 157:487–488, 1992

Silva P, Brown, RS, Epstein FH: Adaptation to potassium. Kidney Int 11:466–475, 1977

Simpson JB, Routtenberg A: The subfornical organ and carbachol induced drinking. Brain Res 45:135–152, 1972

Simpson JB, Routtenberg A: Subfornical organ: site of drinking elicitation by angiotensin-II. Science 181:1172–1175, 1973

Simpson JB, Epstein AN, Camardo JS : Localization of receptors for dipsogenic action of angiotensin II in the subfornical organ of rat. J Comp Physiol Psychol 92:581–608, 1978

Singer SJ, Nicolson GL: The fluid mosaic model of the structure of membranes. Science 175:720–731, 1972

Singh S, Padi MH, Bullard H, et al: Water intoxication in psychiatric patients. Br J Psychiatry 146:127–131, 1985

Skinner BF: Superstitious activity under fixed interval reinforcement. J Exp Psychol 38:168–172, 1948

Sklar AH, Schrier RW: Central nervous system mediators of vasopressin release. Physiol Rev 63:1243–1280, 1983

Skou JC: The influence of some cations on the adenosine triphosphatase from peripheral nerves. Biochim Biophys Acta 23:394–401, 1957

Sladek CD, Armstrong WE: Effect of neurotransmitters and neuropeptides on vasopressin release, in Vasopressin: Principles and Properties. Edited by Gash DM, Boer GJ. New York, Plenum, 1987, pp 275–333

Sleeper FH: Investigation of polyuria in schizophrenia. Am J Psychiatry 91:1019–1031, 1935

Sleeper FH, Jellinek EM: A comparative physiologic, psychologic, and psychiatric study of polyuric and nonpolyuric schizophrenic patients. J Nerv Ment Dis 83:557–563, 1936

Smith RW, McCann SM: Increased and decreased water intake in the rat with hypothalamic lesions, in Thirst. Edited by Wayner MJ. New York, Macmillan, 1964, pp 381–392

Smith WO, Clark ML: Self-induced water intoxication in schizophrenic patients. Am J Psychiatry 137:1055–1060, 1980

Smitt M: Influence of hepatic portal receptors on hypothalamic feeding and satiety centers. Am J Physiol 225:1089–1095, 1973

Snyder SH: Drug and neurotransmitter receptors in the brain. Science 224:22–31, 1984

Southard EE: On the topographical distribution of cortex lesions and anomalies in dementia praecox, with some account of their functional significance. Am J Insanity 71:603–671, 1915

Spielman WS, Davis JO: The renin-angiotensin system and aldosterone secretion during sodium depletion in the rat. Circ Res 35:615–624, 1974

Sprecher H: The metabolism of (n-3) and (n-6) fatty acids and the oxygenation by platlet cyclooxygenase and lipooxygenase. Prog Lipid Res 25:19–28, 1986

Stahl SM: Peripheral models for the study of neurotransmitter receptors in man. Psychopharmacol Bull 21:663–671, 1985

Stam J, Van Oers MHJ, Verbeeten B: Recovery after central pontine myelinolysis. J Neurol 231:52–53, 1984

Stein L, Seifter J: Muscarinic synapses in the hypothalamus. Am J Physiol 202:751–756, 1962

Steller U, Koschorek F, Strenge H: Cerebellar ataxia with recovery related to central pontine myelinolysis. J Neurol 235:379–381, 1988

Sterns RH: Severe symptomatic hyponatremia: treatment and outcome. Ann Intern Med 1987; 107:656–664, 1987

Sterns RH: The management of symptomatic hyponatremia. Semin Nephrol 10:503–514, 1990

Sterns RH: "Slow" correction of hyponatremia: a break with tradition? Kidney 23:1–4, 1991

Sterns RH, Spital A: Disorders of water balance, in Fluids and Electrolytes. Edited by Kokko JP, Tannen RL. Philadelphia, PA, WB Saunders, 1990, pp 139–194

Sterns RH, Riggs JE, Schochet SS Jr: Osmotic demyelination syndrome following correction of hyponatremia. N Engl J Med 3314:1535–1542, 1986

Sterns RH, Thomas DJ, Herndon RM: Brain dehydration and neurologic deterioration after rapid correction of hyponatremia. Kidney Int 35: 69–75, 1989

Sterns RJ, Baer J, Eberson S, et al: Organic osmolytes in acute hyponatremia. Am J Physiol 264:F833–F836, 1993

Stevens JD: The distribution of phospholipid fractions in the red cell membrane of schizophrenics. Schizophr Bull 6:60–61, 1972

Strauss MB: Body Water in Man: The Acquisition and Maintenance of Body Fluids. Boston, MA, Little, Brown, 1957

Stricker EM: Extracellular fluid volume and thirst. Am J Physiol 211: 232–238, 1966

Stricker EM: Drinking by rats after lateral hypothalamic lesions: a new look at the lateral hypothalamic syndrome. J Comp Physiol Psychol 90:127–143, 1976

Stricker EM: The renin-angiotensin system and thirst: some unanswered questions. Fed Proc 37: 2704–2710, 1978

Stricker EM: Thirst and sodium appetite after colloid treatments in rats. J Comp Physiol Psychol 95:1–25, 1981

Stricker EM, Swerdloff AF, Zigmond MJ: Intrahypothalamic injections of kainic acid produce feeding and drinking deficits in rats. Brain Res 158:470–473, 1978

Stricker EM, Vagnuci AH, McDonald RH: Renin and aldosterone secretions during hypovolemia in rats: relation to NaCl intake. Am J Physiol 237:R45–R51, 1979

Suddath RL, Casanova MF, Goldberg TE, et al: Temporal lobe pathology in schizophrenia: a quantitative magnetic resonance imaging study. Am J Psychiatry 146:464–472, 1989a

Suddath RL, Foote M, Godleski L, et al: MRI of polydipsia-hyponatremia. 1989 CME Syllabus & Proceedings Summary, 142nd Annual Meeting of the American Psychiatric Association, San Francisco, CA, May 6–11, 1989b, p 158

Suddath RL, Christison GW, Torrey EF, et al: Anatomical abnormalities in the brains of monozygotic twins discordant for schizophrenia. N Engl J Med 322:789–794, 1990

Summy-Long J, WB Severs: Angiotensin and thirst: studies with a converting enzyme inhibitor and a receptor antagonist. Life Sci 15: 569–582, 1974

Suzuki M, Takeuchi O, Mori I, et al: Syndrome of inappropriate secretion of antidiuretic hormone associated with schizophrenia. Biol Psychiatry 31:1057–1061, 1992

Swanson LW, Sawchenko PE: Paraventricular nucleus: a site for the integration of neuroendocrine and autonomic mechanisms. Neuroendocrinology 31:410–417, 1980

Swanson LW, Sawchenko PE: Hypothalamic integration: organization of the paraventricular and supraoptic nuclei. Annu Rev Neurosci 6: 269–324, 1983

Swanson LW, Kucharczyk J, Mogenson GJ: Autoradiographic evidence for pathways from the medial preoptic area to the midbrain involved in the drinking response to angiotensin II. J Comp Neurol 178: 645–660, 1978

Swayze VW 2nd, Andreasen NC, Alliger RJ, et al: Subcortical and temporal structures in affective disorder and schizophrenia: a magnetic resonance imaging study. Biol Psychiatry 31:221–240, 1992

Sweadner KJ: Two molecular forms of (Na$^+$+ K$^+$)-stimulated ATPase in brain. Separation and difference in affinity for strophanthidine. J Biol Chem 254:6060–6067, 1979

Sweadner KJ: Isozymes of the (Na$^+$+ K$^+$)-ATPase. Biochim Biophys Acta 988:185–220, 1989

Sweadner KJ, Goldin SM: Active transport of sodium and potassium ions: mechanism, function and regulation. N Engl J Med 302:777–783, 1980

Takayanagi R, Tanaka I, Maki M, et al: Effects of changes in water-sodium balance on levels of atrial natriuretic factor messenger RNA and peptide in rats. Life Sci 36:1843–1848, 1985

Tallis GA: Hyponatremia in psychiatric patients. Med J Aust 150:151–153, 1989

Tamir H, Mahadik SP, Rapport MM: Fractionation of synaptic plasma membranes with diatrizoate. Anal Biochem 76:634–647, 1976

Tanaka R, Teruya A: Lipid dependence of activity-temperature relationship of (Na$^+$+, K$^+$)-activated ATPase. Biochim Biophys Acta 323:584–591, 1973

Tandon R, Mazzara C, DeQuardo J, et al: Dexamethasone suppression test in schizophrenia: relationship to symptomatology, ventricular enlargement and outcome. Biol Psychiatry 29:953–964, 1991

Tang M, Falk JL: Sar-Ala angiotensin II blocks renin-angiotensin but not beta-adrenergicdipsogens. Pharmacol Biochem Behav 2:401–408, 1974

Tanneau R, Garre M, Pennec YL, et al: Brain damage and spontaneous correction of hyponatremia. Lancet 2:1031–1032, 1988

Teitelbaum P, Epstein AN: The lateral hypothalamic syndrome: recovery of feeding and drinking after lateral hypothalamic lesions. Psychol Rev 69:74–90, 1962

Thompson AJ, Brown MM, Swash M, et al: Autopsy validation of MRI in central pontine myelinolysis. Neuroradiology 30:175–177, 1988

Thompson CJ, Baylis PH: Osmoregulation of thirst. J Endocr 155–157, 1988

Thompson CJ, Burd JM, Baylis PH: Acute suppression of plasma vasopressin and thirst after drinking in hypernatremic humans. Am J Physiol 252:R1138–R1142, 1987

Thompson CJ, Edwards CRW, Baylis PH: Osmotic and non-osmotic regulation of thirst and vasopressin secretion in patients with compulsive water drinking. Clin Endocrinol (Oxf) 35:221–228, 1991

Thompson DS, Hutton JT, Stears JC, et al: Computerized tomography in the diagnosis of central and extrapontine myelinolysis. Arch Neurol 38:243–246, 1981

Thompson PD, Miller D, Gledhill RF, et al: Magnetic resonance imaging in central pontine myelinolysis. J Neurol Neurosurg Psychiatry 52: 675–677, 1989

Thrasher TN, Simpson JB, Ramsay DJ: Lesions of the subfornical organ block angiotensin-induced drinking in the dog. Neuroendocrinology 35:68–72, 1982

Thurston JH, Hauhart RE, Mallinedrodt E: Brain amino acids decrease in chronic hyponatremia and rapid correction causes brain dehydration: possible clinical significance. Life Sci 1987; 40:2539–2542, 1987

Tien R, Arieff AI, Kucharzyk W, et al: Hyponatremic encephalopathy: is central pontine myolinolysis a component? Am J Med 92:513–522, 1992

Tinker R, Anderson MG, Anand P, et al: Pontine myelinolysis presenting with acute parkinsonism as a sequel of corrected hyponatremia. J Neurol Neurosurg Psychiatry 53:87–89, 1990

Tombaugh TN, McIntyre NJ: The Mini-Mental State examination: a comprehensive review. J Am Geriatr Soc 40:922–933, 1992

Tomlinson BE, Pierides AM, Bradley WG: Central pontine myelinolysis: two cases with associated electrolyte disturbance. Q J Med 45: 373–386, 1976

Totterdell S, Smith AD: Convergence of hippocampal and dopaminergic input onto identified neurons in the nucleus accumbens of the rat. J Chem Neuroanat 2:285–289, 1989

Trabert W, Huber G, Bellaire W, et al: Klinische und computertomographische verlaufsuntersuchung einer selbstinduzierten wasserintoxikation. Nervenarzt 58:637–639, 1987

Turker RK: A general review of angiotensin peptides and 8-substituted analogs of angiotensin II, in The Physiology of Thirst and Sodium Appetite. Edited by de Caro G, Epstein AN, Massi M. New York, Plenum, 1986, pp 205–212

Umbricht DSG, Saltz B, Pollack S, et al: Polydipsia and tardive dyskinesia in chronic psychiatric patients—Related disorders? Am J Psychiatry 150:1536–1538, 1993

Unger T, Ganten D, Ludvig G, et al: The brain-renin-angiotensin system: update, in The Physiology of Thirst and Sodium Appetite. Edited by de Caro G, Epstein AN, Massi M. New York, Plenum, 1986, pp 123–133

Urano A, Kobayash H: Effects of noradrenaline and dopamine injected into the supraoptic nucleus on urine flow rate in hydrated rats. Exp Neurol 60:140–150, 1978

Urayama O, Sweadner KJ: Quabain sensitivity of the alpha 3 isozyme of rat (Na$^+$+ K$^+$)-ATPase. Biochim Biophys Res Commun 156:796–800, 1988

Urayama O, Shutt H, Sweadner KJ: Identification of three isozyme proteins of the catalytic subunit of (Na$^+$+ K$^+$)-ATPase in rat brain. J Biol Chem 264:8271–8280, 1989

Utzon NP, Dessau RB: Psychogenic polydipsia: pronounced cerebral edema after exaggerated consumption of boiled water. Ugeskr Laeger 153:723–724, 1991

Valenstein ESI: Invited comment: Electrical stimulation and hypothalamic function: historical perspective, in The Neuropsychology of Thirst. Edited by Epstein AN, Kissileff HR, Stellar E. New York, Wiley, 1973, pp 155–161

Valenstein ES, Cox VC, Kakolewski JW: Modification of motivated behavior by electrical stimulation of the hypothalamus. Science 159: 1119–1121, 1968

Vance WB: Observations on the role of salivary secretions in the regulation of food and fluid intake in the white rat. Psychol Monogr 79: (5, Whole No. 598), 1965

van Deenen, LLM: Some structural and dynamic aspects of lipids in biological membranes. Ann N Y Acad Sci 137:717–730, 1966

van Kammen DP, Mann LS, Sternberg DE, et al: Dopamine-beta-hydroxylase activity and homovanillic acid in spinal fluid of schizophrenics with brain atrophy. Science 220:974–977, 1983

van Kammen DP, Yao JK, Goetz K: Polyunsaturated fatty acids, prostaglandins and schizophrenia. Ann NY Acad Sci 559:411–424, 1989

Van Reeth O, Decaux G: Rapid correction of hyponatremia with urea may protect against brain damage in rats. Clin Sci 77:351–355, 1989

Varon S, Manthorpe M, Davis GE, et al: Growth factors, in Functional Recovery in Neurological Disease, Advances in Neurology, Vol. 47. Edited by Waxman SG. New York, Raven, 1988, pp 493–521

Veldhuis JD, Johnson ML: An overview of computer algorithms for deconvolution-based assessment of in vivo neuroendocrine secretory events. Biotechniques 8:634–639, 1990

Veldhuis JD, Carlson ML, Johnson ML: The pituitary gland secretes in bursts: appraising the nature of glandular secretory impulses by simultaneous multiple-parameter deconvolution of plasma hormone concentrations. Proc Natl Acad Sci U S A 84:7686–7690, 1987

Verbalis JG: Hyponatraemia. Baillieres Clin Endocrinol Metab 3:499–529, 1989

Verbalis JG, Dohanics J: Vasopressin and oxytocin secretion in chronically hyposmolar rats. Am J Physiol 261:R1028–R1038, 1991

Verbalis JG, Drutarosky MD: Adaptation to chronic hypoosmolality in rats. Kidney Int 34:351–360, 1988

Verbalis JG, Gullans SR: Hyponatremia causes large sustained reductions in brain content of multiple organic osmolytes in rats. Brain Res 567:274–282, 1991a

Verbalis JG, Gullans SR: Rapid correction of chronic hyponatremia produces differential effects on brain osmolyte and electrolyte reaccumulation in rats. J Am Soc Nephrol 2:769, 1991b

Verbalis JG, Martinez AJ: Neurological and neuropathological sequelae of correction of chronic hyponatremia. Kidney Int 39:1274–1282, 1991

Veress AT, Sonnenberg H: Right atrial appendectomy reduces the renal response to acute hypervolemia in the rat. Am J Physiol 247:R610–R613, 1984

Verghese C, DeLeon J, Simpson GM: Clozapine treatment of polydipsia: a prolactin connection (Letter). J Clin Psychopharmacol 12:218, 1992

Verghese C, DeLeon J, Simpson GM: Neuroendocrine factors influencing polydipsia in psychiatric patients: an hypothesis. Neuropsychopharmacology 9:157–166, 1993

Verney EB: The antidiuretic hormone and the factors which determine its release. Proc R Soc Lond B Biol Sci 135:27–106, 1947

Vestergaard P, Leverett R: Constancy of urinary creatinine excretion. J Lab Clin Med 51:211–218, 1958

Vieweg WVR: Behavioral approaches to polydipsia. Biol Psychiatry 34:125–127, 1993

Vieweg WVR: Treatment strategies in the polidipsia-hyponatremia syndrome. J Clin Psychiatry 55:154–160, 1994

Vieweg WVR, David JJ: Polyuria and schizophrenia. Psychiatry Res 17:329–330, 1986

Vieweg WVR, Godleski LS: Carbamazepine and hyponatremia. Am J Psychiatry 145:1323–1324, 1988a

Vieweg WVR, Godleski LS: Hyponatremia and atrial natriuretic peptide secretion in patients with vasopressin-induced antidiuresis. Am J Med 85:594, 1988b

Vieweg WVR, Karp BI: Severe hyponatremia in the polydipsia–hyponatremia syndrome J Clin Psychiatry 55(8):355–361, 1994

Vieweg WVR, Rowe WT, David JJ, et al: Evaluation of patients with self-induced water intoxication and schizophrenic disorders (SIWIS). J Nerv Ment Dis 172:552–555, 1984a

256   WATER BALANCE IN SCHIZOPHRENIA

Vieweg WVR, Rowe WT, David JJ, et al: Hyposthenuria as a marker for
self-induced water intoxication and schizophrenic disorders. Am
J Psychiatry 141:1258–1260, 1984b

Vieweg WVR, Rowe WT, David JJ, et al: The "Mini-Mental State" in the
syndrome of self-induced water intoxication and schizophrenic disorders (SIWIS): a pilot study. Int J Psychiatry Med 14:347–359, 1984c

Vieweg V, Rowe W, David J, et al: Hyposthenuria as a marker for self-
induced water intoxication and schizophrenic disorders. Am J Psychiatry 141:1258–1260, 1984d

Vieweg WVR, David JJ, Rowe WT, et al: Death from self-induced water
intoxication and schizophrenic disorders (SIWIS). J Nerv Ment Dis
173:161–165, 1985a

Vieweg WVR, David JJ, Rowe WT, et al: Psychogenic polydipsia and water intoxication—concepts that have failed. Biol Psychiatry 20:
1308–1320, 1985b

Vieweg WVR, Rowe WT, David JJ, et al: Patterns of urinary excretion
among patients with self-induced water intoxication and psychosis
(SIWIP). Psychiatry Res 15:71–79, 1985c

Vieweg WVR, Rowe WT, David JJ, et al: Possible ameliorating effect of
captopril treatment and hyperosmolar coma in a patient with psychosis, intermittent hyponatremia, and polydipsia. Psychiatr Hosp
16:183–186, 1985d

Vieweg WVR, Rowe WT, David JJ, et al: Oral sodium chloride in the management of schizophrenic patients with self-induced water intoxication. J Clin Psychiatry 46:16–19, 1985e

Vieweg WVR, David JJ, Glick JL, et al: Polyuria among patients with psychosis. Schizophr Bull 12:739–743, 1986a

Vieweg WVR, David JJ, Rowe WT, et al: Correlation of cigarette-induced
serum nicotine levels and arginine vasopressin determinations in the
syndrome of self-induced water intoxication and psychosis (SIWIP).
Can J Psychiatry 31:108–111, 1986b

Vieweg WVR, David JJ, Rowe WT, et al: Diurnal variation of urinary excretion for patients with psychosis, intermittent hyponatremia, and
polydipsia (PIP syndrome). Biol Psychiatry 21:1031–1042, 1986c

Vieweg WVR, David JJ, Rowe WT, et al: Hypocalcemia: an additional complication of the syndrome of self-induced water intoxication and psychosis (SIWIP). Psychiatr Med 4:291–297, 1986d

Vieweg WVR, Rowe WT, David JJ, et al: Self-induced water intoxication
and psychosis (SIWIP): subcategory of the syndrome of inappropriate antidiuresis (SIAD). Psychiatr Med 4:277–290, 1986e

Vieweg WVR, Godleski L, Yank G: Diurnal weight gain as an index of polyuria and hyponatremia among chronically psychotic patients. Neuroendocrinol Lett 9:218, 1987a

Vieweg WVR, Rowe WT, David JJ, et al: Self-induced water intoxication and psychosis (SIWIP): Subcategory of the syndrome of inappropriate antidiuresis (SIAD). Psychiatr Med 4:277–290, 1987b

Vieweg V, Glick JL, Herring S, et al: Absence of carbamazepine-induced hyponatremia among patients also given lithium. Am J Psychiatry 144:943–947, 1987c

Vieweg WVR, David JJ, Rowe WT, et al: Correlation of parameters of urinary excretion with serum osmolality among patients with psychosis, intermittent hyponatremia, and polydipsia. Psychiatr Med 6: 81–97, 1988a

Vieweg WVR, David JJ, Rowe WT, et al: Nomograms of polyuria for men and women with psychosis, intermittent hyponatremia, and polydipsia (PIP syndrome). Psychiatr Med 6:29–40, 1988b

Vieweg WVR, Godleski LS, Goldman F, et al: Abnormal diurnal weight gain among chronically psychotic patients compared to a control population. Acta Psychiatr Scand 78:169–171, 1988c

Vieweg WVR, Godleski LS, Graham P, et al: Abnormal diurnal weight gain among long-term patients with schizophrenic disorders. Schizophr Res 1:67–71, 1988d

Vieweg WVR, Godleski LS, Hundley PL, et al: Diurnal weight gain as an index of polyuria and hyponatremia among chronically psychotic patients. Psychiatr Med 6:23–28, 1988e

Vieweg WVR, Godleski LS, Hundley PL, et al: Lithium, polyuria, and abnormal diurnal weight gain in psychosis. Acta Psychiatr Scand 78: 510–514, 1988f

Vieweg WVR, Godleski LS, Pavalonis DL, et al: Abnormal diurnal weight gain in chronic psychosis without seasonal change. Neuropsychobiology 19:176–179, 1988g

Vieweg WVR, Hundley PL, Godleski LS, et al: Diurnal weight gain as a predictor of serum sodium concentration among patients with psychosis, intermittent hyponatremia, and polydipsia (PIP syndrome). Psychiatry Res 26:305–312, 1988h

Vieweg WVR, Hundley PL, Godleski LS, et al: Similarity of patterns of urine excretion among nonpolyuric and polyuric patients with thought disorders. Schizophr Res 1:295–298, 1988i

Vieweg WVR, Robertson GL, Godleski LS, et al: Diurnal variation in water homeostasis among schizophrenic patients subject to water intoxication. Schizophr Res 1:351–357, 1988j

Vieweg WVR, Weiss NM, David JJ, et al: Treatment of psychosis, intermittent hyponatremia, and polydipsia (PIP syndrome) with lithium and phenytoin. Biol Psychiatry 23:25–30, 1988k

Vieweg WVR, Wilkinson EC, David JJ, et al: The use of demeclocycline in the treatment of patients with psychosis, intermittent hyponatremia, and polydipsia (PIP syndrome). Psychiatr Q 59:62–68, 1988l

Vieweg WVR, Godleski LS, Graham P, et al: Diurnal weight gain in chronic psychosis. Schizophr Bull 15:501–506, 1989a

Vieweg WVR, Godleski LS, Harrington DP, et al: Antipsychotic drugs, lithium, carbamazepine, and abnormal diurnal weight gain in psychosis. Neuropsychopharmacology 2:39–43, 1989b

Vieweg WVR, Godleski LS, Hundley PL, et al: Failure of antipsychotic drug dose to explain abnormal diurnal weight gain among 129 chronically psychotic inpatients. Prog Neuropsychopharmacol Biol Psychiatry 13:709–723, 1989c

Vieweg WVR, Godleski LS, Hundley PL, et al: Survey of diurnal weight gain and urine volume in chronic schizophrenia. Can J Psychiatry 34:779–784, 1989d

Vieweg WVR, Godleski LS, Mitchell M, et al: Abnormal diurnal weight gain among chronically psychotic patients contrasted with acutely psychotic patients and normals. Psychol Med 19:105–109, 1989e

Vieweg WVR, Godleski LS, Pulliam WR, et al: Development of water dysregulation during Arieti's third stage of schizophrenia? Biol Psychiatry 26:775–780, 1989f

Vieweg WVR, Godleski LS, Shannon C, et al: Normalization of abnormal diurnal weight gain among chronically psychotic geriatric patients. Is abnormal diurnal weight gain a risk factor in chronic psychosis? J Nerv Ment Dis 177:542–545, 1989g

Vieweg WVR, Godleski LS, Shannon C, et al: Diurnal weight gain among patients with mental retardation. Am J Ment Retard 93:558–565, 1989h

Vieweg WVR, Carey RM, Godleski LS, et al: The syndrome of psychosis, intermittent hyponatremia, and polydipsia: evidence for diurnal volume expansion. Psychiatr Med 8:135–144, 1990a

Vieweg WVR, Godleski LS, Graham P, et al: Abnormal diurnal weight gain among institutionalized patients with manic-depressive spectrum disorders. Psychiatr Med 8:129–134, 1990b

Vieweg WVR, Harrington DP, Leadbetter RA, et al: Prediction of serum sodium based on diurnal weight gain among schizophrenics subject to water intoxication. Psychiatrie & Psychobiologie 5:265–267, 1990c

Vieweg WVR, Harrington DP, Westerman PS, et al: Seasonal stability of water balance among schizophrenic patients subject to water intoxication. Prog Neuropsychopharmacol Biol Psychiatry 14:215–222, 1990d

Vieweg WVR, Godleski LS, Graham P, et al: The link between drinking and weight gain in psychosis. Psychosomatics 32:52–57, 1991a

Vieweg V, Veldhuis J, Leadbetter R, et al: Cigarette use and hyponatremia in schizophrenic patients. Am J Psychiatry 148:688–689, 1991b

Vieweg WVR, Pandurangi AK, Pelonero AL: Estimating daily urine volume in chronic psychosis. Schizophr Res 8:89–91, 1992a

Vieweg WVR, Veldhuis JD, Carey RM: Temporal pattern of renin and aldosterone secretion in men: effects of sodium balance. Am J Physiol 262:F871–F877, 1992b

Vieweg V, Lombana A, Lewis R: Hyper- and hyponatremia among geropsychiatric inpatients. J Geriatr Psychiatry Neurol 1993

Vieweg V, Pandurangi A, Levinson J, et al: The consulting psychiatrist and the polydipsia–hyponatremia syndrome in schizophrenia. Int J Psychiatry Med 24:275–303, 1994

Vlajkovic S, Zwetnow NN, Thomas KA, et al: Magnetic resonance imaging of water intoxication: an experimental study in dogs. Acta Radiol Suppl 369:353–355, 1986

von den Velden R: Die nierenwirkung von hypophysenextrakten beim menschen. Berl Munch Tierarztl Wochenschr 1:2083–2090, 1913

Waddington JL, Youssef HA: Late onset involuntary movements in schizophrenia: relationship of tardive dyskinesia to intellectual impairment and negative symptoms. Br J Psychiatry 149:616–620, 1986

Wagman AM, Heinrichs DW, Carpenter WT Jr: Deficit and nondeficit forms of schizophrenia: neuropsychological evaluation. Psychiatry Res 22:319–330, 1987

Wainwright PE: Do essential fatty acids play a role in brain and behavioral development. Neurosci Behav Rev 16:193–205, 1992

Wakerly JB, Lincoln DW: Phasic discharge of antidromically identified units in the paraventricular nucleus of the hypothalamus. Brain Res 25:192–194, 1971

Waldman AJ: Neuroanatomic/neuropathologic correlates in schizophrenia (Review Article). South Med J 85:907–916, 1992

Walker JV, Englander RN: Central pontine myelinolysis following rapid correction of hyponatremia in an alcoholic. Am J Kidney Dis 12:531–533, 1988

Wallace M, Singer G: Schedule induced behavior: a review of its generality, determinants and pharmacological data. Pharmacol Biochem Behav 5:483–490, 1976

Wallace M, Singer G, Wayner MJ, et al: Adjunctive behavior in humans during game playing. Physiol Behav 14:651–654, 1975

Wallace M, Singer G, Finlay J, et al: The effect of 6–OHDA lesions of the nucleus acumbens septum on schedule-induced drinking, wheel running and corticosterone levels in the rat. Pharmacol Biochem Behav 18:129–136, 1983

Walsh LL, Grossman SP: Zona incerta lesions: disruption of regulatory water intake. Physiol Behav 11:885–887, 1973

Walsh LL, Grossman SP: Zona incerta lesions impair osmotic but not hypovolemic thirst. Physiol Behav 16:211–215, 1976

Walsh LL, Grossman SP: Dissociation of responses to extracellular thirst stimuli following zona incerta lesions. Pharmacol Biochem Behav 8:409–416, 1978

Webb WL, Gehi M: Electrolyte and fluid imbalance: neuropsychiatric manifestations. Psychosomatics 22:199–203, 1981

Weinberger DR: Implications of normal brain development for the pathogenesis of schizophrenia. Arch Gen Psychiatry 44:660–669, 1987

Weinberger DR, Bigelow LB, Kleinman JE, et al: Cerebral ventricular enlargement in chronic schizophrenia: an association with poor response to treatment. Arch Gen Psychiatry 37:11–13, 1980

Weindl A, Sofroniew M: Neuroanatomical pathways related to vasopressin, in Current topics in neuroendocrinology. Edited by Ganten D, Pfaff D. Berlin, Springer-Verlag, 1985

Weir JF, Larson EE, Rowntree LG: Studies in diabetes insipidus, water balance, and water intoxication: study I. Arch Intern Med 29:306–330, 1922

Weisberg LS: Pseudohyponatremia: a reappraisal. Am J Med 86:315–318, 1989

Weiss ML: Sodium appetite induced by sodium depletion is suppressed by intracerebroventricular captopril, in The Physiology of Thirst and Sodium Appetite. Edited by de Caro G, Epstein AN, Massi M. New York, Plenum Press, 1986, pp 405–411

Weissman JD, Weissman BM: Pontine myelinolysis and delayed encephalopathy following rapid correction of acute hyponatremia. Arch Neurol 46:926–927, 1989

Weitzman RE, Kleeman CR: The clinical physiology of water metabolism: part I: the physiologic regulation of arginine vasopressin secretion and thirst. West J Med 131:373–400, 1979

Whittaker VP: Some properties of synaptic membranes isolated from the central nervous system. Ann N Y Acad Sci 137:982–998, 1966

Whittam R, Wheeler KP: Transport across cell membranes. Annu Rev Physiol 32:21–60, 1970

Wiesel F-A: Altered transport of tyrosine across the blood-brain barrier in patients with schizophrenia, in International Congress Series, Vol 968. Edited by Racagni G, Brunello N, Fukuda T. Amsterdam, Excerpta Medica, 1991, pp 337–340

Williams DR, Teitelbaum P: Some observations on the starvation resulting from lateral hypothalamic lesions. J Comp Physiol Psychol 52: 458–465, 1959

Winkler SS, Thomasson DM, Sherwood K, et al: Regional T2 and sodium concentration estimates in the normal human brain by Sodium–23 MRI imaging at 1.5T. J Comput Assist Tomogr 13:561–566, 1989

Winslow JT, Hastings N, Carter CS, et al: A role for central vasopressin in pair bonding in monogamous prairie voles. Nature 365:545–548, 1993

Wise RA: Plasticity of hypothalamic motivational systems. Science 162: 377–379, 1969

Wittert GA, Or HK, Livesey JH, et al: Vasopressin, corticotrophin-releasing factor, and pituitary adrenal responses to acute cold stress in normal humans. J Clin Endocrinol Metab 75:750–755, 1992

Wood RJ, Maddison S, Rolls ET, et al: Drinking in the rhesus monkey: roles of pre-systemic and systemic factors in drinking control. J Comp Physiol Psychol 94:1135–1148, 1980

Wood RJ, Rolls ET, Rolls BJ: Physiological mechanisms for thirst in the non-human primate. Am J Physiol 242:423, 1982

Woodbury JW: The cell membrane: ionic and potential gradients and active transport, in Medical Physiology and Biophysics. Edited by Ruch TC, Fulton JF. Philadelphia, PA, WB Saunders, 1974, pp 2–30

Wright DG, Laureno R, Victor M: Pontine and extrapontine myelinolysis. Brain 102:361–385, 1979

Wszolek ZK, McComb RD, Pfeiffer RF, et al: Pontine and extrapontine myelinolysis following liver transplantation. Transplantation 48: 1006–1012, 1989

Zegers de Beyl D, Flament-Durand J, Borenstein S, et al: Ocular bobbing and myoclonus in central pontine myelinolysis. J Neurol Neurosurg Psychiatr 46:564–565, 1983

Zerbe R, Stropes L, Robertson G: Vasopressin function in the syndrome of inappropriate antidiuresis. Annu Rev Med 31:315–327, 1980

Zipursky RB, Lim KO: Evidence for diffuse gray matter abnormalities in schizophrenia, in Society for Neuroscience Abstracts: Society for Neuroscience 20th Annual Meeting, St Louis, MO, October 28–November 2, 1990, p 1349

Zubenko GS, Altesman RI, Cassidy JW, et al: Disturbances of thirst and water homeostasis in patients with affective illness. Am J Psychiatry 141:436–437, 1984

Zubenko GS: Water homeostasis in psychiatric patients. Biol Psychiatry 22:121–125, 1987

Index

*Page numbers printed in **bold** type refer to tables or figures.*

Grooming, 141
Group psychotherapy,
 polydipsic-hyponatremic
 patients and, 36–37
Guanosine triphosphate, 97

Hallucinations, 141
Haloperidol, 7, 12, 82
Hemorrhage, thirst and, 63
Hippocampal lesions, 144–145
Histamine injections, 83
Hoarding, 138–139, 141, 142
Homovanillic acid (HVA), 130
Hospitalization, duration, 150,
 154–155, 159–160
HVA. *See* Homovanillic acid
Hydration, body function of,
 54–55
Hydronephrosis, 33
Hydrostatic pressure, 89–90
Hypercalciuria, 34
Hyperdipsia, 72
Hypernatremia, thirst and, 63
Hyperphagia, 72
Hyperprolactinemia, diuresis
 and, 12
Hypersexuality, 140, 141–142
Hypervolemic hyponatremia,
 45–47
Hypocalcemia, 34
Hypodipsia, zona incerta
 lesions and, 73
Hyponatremia. *See also*
 Polydipsia-hyponatremia
 syndrome; Water
 intoxication
 acute versus chronic,
 177–178

antidiuresis sodium
 concentration
 relationship, **30**
brain adaptation to,
 167–170
community care, 197–198
differential diagnosis, 185
etiology in psychiatric
 patients, 101–103
euvolemic, 45–47
extended care, 194–197
hypervolemic, 45–47
hypovolemic, 45–47
identifying, 182–183
interventions based on
 weight gain, 192–194
management of, 177–179
mechanism of, **21**
medical sequelae,
 183–185
monitoring procedures,
 187–192
mortality, 166
myelinolysis and,
 170–176
progression to, 184–185
pseudohyponatremia, 46
psychotic exacerbation and
 elevated vasopressin,
 118–120
related complications, **32**
symptoms of, 167
volume state and, 45–47
Hyponatremia (dilutional)
 antipsychotic drug dose
 and, 13
 hyposthenuria and, 31
 major factors leading to, **21**

Mean urine creatinine
concentration (MUCR),
23–24
Medial preoptic area, 74–75
Medical sequelae,
hyponatremia and
polydipsia, 183–185
Medication interventions,
196–197
Megacystis, 33
Membrane. *See* Plasma
membrane
Mental retardation, water
imbalance in, 34–35
Methionine-enkephalin, 84
Methylphenidate, 119–120
Mini-Mental State Exam
(MMSE) scores, 153–157
MMSE. *See* Mini-Mental State
Exam
Molindone, 205
Monitoring procedures,
187–192
Morphine injections, 84
Motor retardation, 141
MRI. *See* Magnetic resonance
imaging
MSS. *See* Mean serum sodium
concentration
MUCR. *See* Mean urine
creatinine concentration
Myelinolysis, 166, 170–177,
203

Na$^+$-K$^+$-ATPase, 98–100
Na$^+$-K$^+$ pump, 90, 95–96,
98–100
Naloxone, 84

Naltrexone, 84, 208, 210
Natriuresis, 50–51, 69
NDWG. *See* Normalized
diurnal weight gain
Negative symptoms,
schizophrenic patient
ratings, 141–143
Nephrectomy, 68, 72
Neuroleptics, 115–116,
205–206
Nicotine, 48–49, 141, 184
Nigrostriatal projections,
70–71
NMR. *See* Nuclear magnetic
resonance spectroscopy
Norepinephrine injections,
82
Normal urine dilution, studies
defining, 18
Normalized diurnal weight
gain (NDWG), 13, 27–31,
34–35, 38
Nuclear magnetic resonance
(NMR) spectroscopy,
132–133
Nucleus medianus, 76, 78–79

Opiate receptors, thirst and,
11
Opioid injections, 84
Oral metering, 59
Oral water loading, effects of,
113. *See also* Fluid intake;
Water loading
Organum vasculosum of the
lamina terminalis and
nucleus medianus, 76–77,
78–79